Allergy and Clinical Immunology: Joint Royal Colleges of Physicians Training Board (JRCPTB)

Azhar ul Haque Sario

Copyright

Azhar.sario@hotmail.co.uk

ORCID: https://orcid.org/0009-0004-8629-830X

LinkedIn: https://www.linkedin.com/in/azharulhaquesario/

Publisher Details Azhar Sario Hungary Author Website: www.linkedin.com/in/azharulhaquesario

Cataloging Data ISBN:

Google Version
978-3-384-80780-9

eBook Version
978-3-384-80781-6

Paperback Version
978-3-384-80782-3

First Edition: 2026 Printed & Distributed by PublishDrive

Contents

The Allergy and Clinical Immunology Training Pathway and Professional Identity

1.1 The Evolution of the Specialty: ACI versus ACLI Pathways

The Great Bifurcation: A Strategic Response

In August 2021, the Joint Royal Colleges of Physicians Training Board (JRCPTB) implemented a curriculum overhaul that fundamentally reshaped our professional landscape. Before this date, the lines were often blurred between "Allergists" and "Immunologists." Today, in 2026, we operate under two distinct, yet deeply symbiotic pathways: Allergy and Clinical Immunology (ACI) and Allergy, Clinical and Laboratory Immunology (ACLI).

This was not merely an administrative rebranding; it was a strategic response to the changing face of disease.

The ACI pathway—the focus of this course—evolved from the former "Allergy" specialty. It was specifically engineered to produce a new breed of "physician of the immune system." Unlike our ACLI colleagues, whose training is heavily weighted toward the leadership, accreditation (ISO15189), and governance of diagnostic laboratories, the ACI physician is forged in the fires of direct patient care.

However, do not mistake this for a simplification of your role. The ACI consultant is not "lab-light"; rather, they are "clinic-heavy." The 2026 curriculum demands that while you may not be calibrating flow cytometers, you must possess the high-level intellectual framework to interpret their outputs with forensic precision.

Drivers of Change: The "Two Epidemics"

Why was this separation necessary? The answer lies in the dual pressures that began to crush the old service models in the early 2020s.

First, the well-documented "Allergy Epidemic" continued its relentless march. By the mid-2020s, the complexity of allergic disease had escalated. We were no longer just seeing simple hay fever; we were managing multi-system anaphylaxis, complex drug desensitizations in cancer patients, and the lifelong management of food allergies in a globalized food supply chain.

Second, and perhaps more critically for the ACI evolution, was the explosion of Secondary Immunodeficiency (SID). Ten years ago, an immunologist primarily saw Primary Immunodeficiencies (PIDs) like CVID or XLA. Today, your clinic list is likely dominated by patients from other specialties.

The Hematology Interface: Patients on CAR-T cell therapies or rituximab who have been left with zero B-cells.

The Neurology Interface: MS patients on B-cell depleting agents requiring long-term immunoglobulin replacement.

The Rheumatology Interface: Patients on complex biologics who present with bizarre, opportunistic fungal infections.

The ACI pathway was built to handle this volume. It creates a clinician who can sit in a multidisciplinary team (MDT) meeting with oncologists and renal physicians, guiding the immunological safety of their treatments.

The "Bridge" Identity

The most unique aspect of the ACI pathway in 2026 is its "Bridge" function. You are the interpreter.

Consider a practical example: A patient presents with recurrent pneumonias. An organ-based specialist might order a "screen." The ACLI consultant ensures the lab produces a valid result. But you, the ACI physician, act as the bridge. You interpret that marginal vaccine response in the context of the patient's protein-losing enteropathy. You decide whether the risk of immunoglobulin therapy outweighs the benefit. You translate the "bench" data into a "bedside" plan.

Therefore, while the ACLI trainee sits the FRCPath exams to become a laboratory director, the ACI trainee (you) prepares for the ACICE (Allergy and Clinical Immunology Certificate Examination). This exam tests clinical judgment over assay validation, ensuring you are safe to manage the high-risk uncertainties of acute immunological medicine.

1.2 The Capabilities in Practice (CiPs) Framework and Entrustment

From Checklists to Trust

If the ACI/ACLI split changed what we learn, the CiPs framework revolutionized how we are assessed.

In the old days (pre-2021), medical education was often reductionist. A trainee would "tick a box" to say they had performed a procedure three times, and they were deemed competent. But we all know that doing a lumbar puncture on a calm volunteer is different from doing one on a distressed patient at 3 AM.

The 2026 curriculum relies on Entrustable Professional Activities (EPAs), formalized as Capabilities in Practice (CiPs). This is a move away from "competency" (can you do it?) to "entrustment" (do I trust you to do it alone?).

The currency of your progress is no longer just knowledge; it is the level of supervision you require.

The Hierarchy of Entrustment

Your supervisors (both Clinical and Educational) will assess you on a scale that reflects real-world safety. Understanding these levels is crucial for your progression:

Level 1: You are entrusted to observe only. (The "Fly on the Wall" phase).

Level 2: You can act with direct supervision. The consultant is in the room, watching your hands and listening to your words.

Level 3: You can act with indirect supervision. The consultant is in the building or available by phone within minutes. This is the "safe learner" phase.

Level 4: You are entrusted to act unsupervised. This is the "consultant-ready" standard.

The Critical Progression Point: By the time you complete your training (CCT), you must achieve Level 4 in all Specialty CiPs. This means you can manage a complex anaphylaxis list or run an immunology infusion clinic without needing to check in with a senior.

The Interplay: Generic vs. Specialty CiPs

The curriculum divides your capabilities into two baskets, but in practice, they are woven together.

1. Generic CiPs (The "Doctor" Skills): There are six of these, covering the universal requirements of being a consultant in the UK. They include:

Functioning within NHS systems.

Ethical and legal practice.

Communication and shared decision-making.

Patient safety and Quality Improvement (QI).

Research and data management.

Teaching and supervision.

Why do these matter? Because you cannot be a good immunologist if you are a bad doctor. For instance, Generic CiP 2 (Ethics) is tested every time you have to decide if a patient with severe dementia should receive painful subcutaneous immunoglobulin infusions. The immunology (Specialty CiP) might say "yes, the levels are low," but the ethics (Generic CiP) might say "no, this is not in the patient's best interest."

2. Specialty CiPs (The "Immunologist" Skills): For the ACI pathway, there are six specific high-level outcomes. Let's look at how they manifest in 2026 practice:

Specialty CiP 1 & 2: Managing Services: You aren't just seeing patients; you are designing the clinic. Can you set up a rapid-access drug allergy clinic that meets safety standards?

Specialty CiP 3: Lab Interpretation: As discussed, you must advise colleagues on the limitations of tests. When a GP calls asking why a specific IgE is positive but the patient eats the food fine, you need to explain cross-reactivity (CCD) without sounding like a textbook.

Specialty CiP 4: Liaison Psychiatry of the Immune System: This involves supporting the management of patients across the hospital. It is the "roaming diplomat" role, negotiating with respiratory physicians about asthma biologics or with dermatologists about angioedema.

Assessment: The Holistic Judgment

Finally, you will notice a difference in your Annual Review of Competence Progression (ARCP). We no longer count just the number of workplace-based assessments (WBA). Instead, your Educational Supervisor makes a "holistic judgment" based on the evidence.

They act like a judge in a court case. They look at your Multi-Source Feedback (MSF), your case-based discussions, and your reflections. They ask themselves a single, human question: "If I were the patient, would I trust this trainee to treat me?"

If the answer is "yes, without supervision," you have achieved Level 4.

Conclusion: The 2026 ACI Physician

To conclude this module, the ACI physician of 2026 is a sophisticated hybrid. You are the product of a deliberate educational evolution that split the laboratory leadership (ACLI) from the high-intensity clinical interface (ACI). This separation has allowed you to specialize in the complexities of patient management—navigating the rising tides of allergic disease and secondary immunodeficiency with confidence.

1.3 Assessment Strategy: The ACICE and Workplace-Based Assessments

The Philosophy of Assessment in 2026

Assessment in postgraduate medical training has undergone a radical philosophical shift over the last decade. We have moved away from the "tick-box" culture of the early 2010s toward a holistic model of programmatic assessment. For the Allergy and Clinical Immunology (ACI) trainee in 2026, assessment is no longer just about proving you know a fact; it is about demonstrating you can be trusted to act.

The ACI assessment strategy is built on two pillars:

- The Knowledge Pillar: Rigorous, summative testing via the ACICE.

- The Performance Pillar: Continuous, formative feedback via WPBAs and the MCR, culminating in entrustment decisions.

The ACICE: A Definitive Milestone

The Allergy and Clinical Immunology Certificate Examination (ACICE) represents the intellectual backbone of the specialty. Unlike historical exams that forced clinical trainees to memorize obscure laboratory assays irrelevant to patient care, the ACICE is clinically calibrated.

Distinct Features of the ACICE:

Clinical Focus: The syllabus maps directly to the "Clinical CiPs" (Capabilities in Practice). You might be asked to interpret a complex component-resolved diagnostic report for a peanut-allergic teenager, rather than simply listing the molecular weight of Ara h 2.

Format Evolution: The exam has moved away from traditional long essays. It now heavily utilizes Short Answer Questions (SAQs) and Structured Clinical Scenarios. These test "higher-order" thinking—evaluation and synthesis.

Timing: Passing the ACICE is a critical progression gateway, typically required by the end of ST5 or ST6. It is the signal to the Deanery that you possess the theoretical maturity to transition into the final stages of training.

Scenario Example: Old Style Question: "Describe the mechanism of action of Omalizumab." ACICE Style Scenario: "A 35-year-old severe asthmatic on maintenance oral corticosteroids has failed Omalizumab therapy after 4 months. Their IgE is 450 IU/mL. Outline your step-wise approach to investigating 'non-response,' discussing potential mimics of asthma, adherence issues, and alternative biologic selection (e.g., anti-IL5 vs. anti-IL4Ra) based on their eosinophil/FeNO profile."

Workplace-Based Assessments (WPBAs): The Engine of Growth

While the ACICE tests what you know, WPBAs test what you do. In the 2026 curriculum, these are treated as "learning events," not just hurdles.

The Toolkit:

Case-Based Discussion (CbD): These are retrospective deep-dives. You sit with a consultant and unpack a complex case—for example, a patient with suspected Mast Cell Activation Syndrome (MCAS). The focus is on your clinical reasoning. Why did you order that test? How did you handle the patient's anxiety?

Mini-Clinical Evaluation Exercise (mini-CEX): This is a snapshot of live practice. A supervisor watches you take a history from a patient with drug allergy. They assess your communication, empathy, and focused data gathering in real-time.

Direct Observation of Procedural Skills (DOPS): Critical for ACI skills like immunotherapy administration or skin prick testing.

The MCR and Entrustment: The "ciPs" Revolution

The most significant innovation in recent years is the Multiple Consultant Report (MCR). In the past, a single supervisor might write a report. Now, the MCR aggregates the views of all consultants you work with.

This "triangulation" of evidence is used to sign off on Capabilities in Practice (CiPs). These are high-level outcomes. Instead of ticking off "Can measure blood pressure," a CiP asks: "Can this doctor be trusted to manage an acute anaphylaxis call independently?"

The Entrustment Scale (Level 1–4):

Level 1: Observed only.

Level 2: Act with direct supervision (consultant in the room).

Level 3: Act with indirect supervision (consultant available by phone).

Level 4: Entrusted to act unsupervised. (The goal for CCT).

The Educational Supervisor's Report (ESR) synthesizes this MCR data for the ARCP (Annual Review of Competence Progression) panel. The ARCP panel's job is to verify that the evidence supports the entrustment decisions made by the faculty.

1.4 Regulatory Governance and the Gold Guide

The Architecture of Training

To survive and thrive in UK specialty training, you must understand the machinery that governs your career. You are not just an employee of a hospital trust; you are a trainee within a highly regulated national framework.

Key Players:

The GMC (General Medical Council): The ultimate regulator. They approve the curriculum and issue your CCT (Certificate of Completion of Training). They care about patient safety and standards.

The JRCPTB (Joint Royal Colleges of Physicians Training Board): The managers. They write the curriculum (on behalf of the Federation of Royal Colleges) and manage the ePortfolio system.

The Deanery / NHS England (Workforce, Training and Education): Your local employer and training provider. They organize your rotations and run your ARCP.

The Gold Guide: Your Rulebook

The Gold Guide (Reference Guide for Postgraduate Specialty Training in the UK) is the definitive manual for training. In 2026, understanding this document is a form of self-defense and advocacy.

Crucial Gold Guide Mechanisms:

Less Than Full Time (LTFT): Training is no longer a sprint; it's a marathon. The 2021 curriculum (and subsequent updates) entrenched the right to flexible training. Whether for childcare, health, or "Category 3" (personal choice/wellbeing), LTFT is now a normalized part of ACI culture.

Out of Programme (OOP): ACI is an academic specialty. Many trainees take time out for research (OOPR) to complete a PhD. The Gold Guide dictates how this time counts toward your CCT date.

Transferable Capabilities: If you started in Paediatrics and switched to ACI, the "accreditation of transferable competencies" allows you to count previous experience, potentially shortening your training time.

Entry Pathways and the "Prioritisation" Landscape of 2026

Allergy and Clinical Immunology is a Group 2 Specialty. This means it does not include dual training in General Internal Medicine (GIM). You focus purely on the specialty.

Entry Gates: Recruitment into ACI is fiercely competitive due to the small number of national posts. Candidates enter at the ST3 level (or ST4 equivalent in some structures) from three main feeder streams:

Internal Medicine Training (IMT): Completion of IMT Stage 1 (2 years).

ACCS (Acute Care Common Stem): Acute medicine stream.

Paediatrics: A unique feature of ACI is that it accepts paediatric trainees (Level 1 training). This creates a rich, diverse cohort where adult physicians and paediatricians train side-by-side.

The 2026 Recruitment Reality: A vital update for the 2026 cohort is the impact of the Medical Training (Prioritisation) Bill. As of 2026, recruitment prioritisation protocols have tightened to favor UK medical graduates and those with significant NHS experience during the offer stage.

Why this matters: For an international graduate or a trainee returning from years abroad, understanding these specific 2026 governance changes is critical for application strategy. You must ensure your "Right to Work" and "NHS Experience" evidence is meticulously documented to navigate the prioritisation hierarchy.

The "Alternative Certificate"
For those who have not followed a standard UK training path (e.g., IMT), the 2026 requirements for the "Alternative Certificate" of Core Competence are stringent. You must demonstrate that your experience mirrors the exact CiPs of the IMT curriculum—managing acute unselected take, cardiac arrest leadership, and geriatric care—before you can enter the specialist ACI pathway.

Service Management, Quality Improvement, and Leadership

2.1 Delivering Allergy and Immunology Services

The Strategic Framework: The "Hub and Spoke" Model

In 2026, the "Hub and Spoke" model is no longer just a theoretical recommendation; it is the operational standard for ACI services across the UK. This model addresses the "postcode lottery" of care, ensuring that a patient in a remote coastal village has access to the same expertise as a patient in central London.

The Concept: Imagine a bicycle wheel.

The Hub (Tertiary Centre): This is the teaching hospital. It holds the high-cost, high-risk infrastructure. It concentrates on "low volume, high complexity" cases.

The Spoke (Secondary/Community): These are district general hospitals or community clinics. They handle "high volume, low complexity" cases.

Operational Details (2026 Update): Recent legislative changes have refined this model into two distinct operational flows, particularly for pharmacy and drug delivery which underpins our immunotherapy services:

Model 1 (Hub-to-Spoke-to-Patient): The patient sees you at the local Spoke. You prescribe a complex venom immunotherapy. The Hub prepares this customized treatment in their sterile manufacturing unit and ships it to the Spoke. The patient receives their injection locally. Benefit: Safety is centralized; access is localized.

Model 2 (Hub-to-Patient): For stable patients on subcutaneous immunoglobulin (SCIG) home therapy, the Hub manages the prescription and ships directly to the patient's home, bypassing the Spoke entirely. Benefit: Massive reduction in footfall at local clinics.

Why Leadership Matters Here: A "Hub and Spoke" network does not run on autopilot. It requires an ACI consultant to act as the "Network Lead." You must negotiate Service Level Agreements (SLAs) that define who holds the clinical risk. If a patient reacts to a venom injection at the Spoke, does the liability sit with the administering nurse at the Spoke or the prescribing consultant at the Hub? These governance lines must be drawn explicitly in your operational policies.

Navigating the Money: ICBs and Specialized Commissioning

To deliver a service, you must understand who pays for it. The landscape has shifted significantly between 2024 and 2026.

The Shift to Delegated Commissioning: Previously, NHS England centrally commissioned all specialized services. This was often rigid. As of April 2026, we are seeing the maturation of Integrated Care Boards (ICBs) taking on delegated responsibility for many specialized services.

What this means for you: You can no longer just look to national policies. You must build relationships with your local ICB commissioners. You need to prove that your allergy service aligns with local population health needs.

The "Neighbourhood Health" Focus: The 2026 NHS agenda emphasizes community care. If you want funding for a new drug allergy clinic, don't pitch it as a "prestige high-tech unit." Pitch it as a "community-facing service that keeps patients out of A&E."

Writing the Business Case: You will inevitably need to hire more staff or buy new equipment. This requires a Business Case. This is not a clinical letter; it is a financial pitch.

The Trap: Do not write, "We need a dietitian because patients are waiting too long."

The Solution: Write, "Investing £50,000 in a Band 7 Dietitian will reduce our waiting list by 30%, allowing us to discharge 100 complex food allergy patients back to primary care per year. This saves the Trust £80,000 in unnecessary follow-up appointments."

Key Metric: Return on Investment (ROI). In 2026, financial efficiency is the language of leadership.

Logistics: The Art of the Clinic Template

Efficiency is not about rushing; it is about flow. As a service lead, you design the "Clinic Template"—the schedule that dictates the rhythm of the day.

The "Hot and Cold" Split:

Hot Cases (Urgent): You must reserve slots for anaphylaxis, suspected SCID (Severe Combined Immunodeficiency) in infants, or acute drug reactions awaiting surgery. If you fill your clinic 100% with routine follow-ups, you have no safety valve for emergencies.

Cold Cases (Routine): Long-term urticaria or stable rhinitis. These are prime candidates for "Virtual Wards" or nurse-led telephone clinics.

Triage as a Safety Tool: You cannot see everyone. Effective triage is your shield. In 2026, we increasingly use AI-assisted triage tools to flag "red flag" keywords (e.g., "tongue swelling," "hypotension") in referral letters. However, the Consultant's eye remains the final filter. You must empower your team to reject inappropriate referrals (e.g., "chronic fatigue" with no immunological basis) to protect capacity for those with genuine pathology.

2.2 Multidisciplinary Team (MDT) Leadership

The Team Composition: The "Jazz Ensemble" Analogy

Immunology is systemic. It touches every organ. Therefore, you cannot practice in a silo. You lead an MDT.

Think of an orchestra. It has a rigid script and a conductor. That is not an Allergy MDT. An Allergy MDT is like a jazz ensemble. It is collaborative, improvisational, and the "solo" passes between members depending on the patient's need.

The Specialist Nurse: They are often the true face of the service. They lead the immunotherapy clinics and drug challenges. They are the experts in practical delivery.

The Dietitian: In food allergy, the dietitian is not a support act; they are the lead. Diagnosing a milk allergy is easy; ensuring a child grows and thrives without milk is hard.

The Psychologist: 2026 curriculum emphasizes "Psychodermatology" and anxiety management. A patient with anaphylaxis often suffers from PTSD. The psychologist is the bridge between physical safety and mental freedom.

Leadership Style: Situational Leadership

You cannot lead a Professor of Dermatology the same way you lead a trainee nurse. You must adapt. This is Situational Leadership.

Scenario A: The Code Red (Anaphylaxis)

Context: A patient collapses during a drug challenge.

Style: Directive.

Action: "Nurse A, give IM adrenaline. Nurse B, call 2222. Registrar C, secure the airway."

Why: In a crisis, the team craves clarity, not consultation. You must be the commander.

Scenario B: The Complex Case (Chronic Spontaneous Urticaria)

Context: A patient is failing Omalizumab and is depressed. The team is discussing the next step.

Style: Consultative/Coaching.

Action: "What does the team think? Sarah (Nurse), how is she coping with injections? Mike (Psychologist), is stress a trigger here?"

Why: You do not have all the answers. You need to synthesize the collective intelligence of the room.

Human Factors: Psychological Safety

This is the most critical concept in modern leadership. Psychological Safety is the belief that one will not be punished or humiliated for speaking up with ideas, questions, concerns, or mistakes.

The "Huddle" Example: Before a high-risk drug challenge session (e.g., Aspirin desensitization), you hold a morning huddle.

Bad Leadership: "Here is the list. Get it done."

Good Leadership: "Team, we have a complex case in Bed 3. I am worried about his asthma control. Does anyone else see any red flags before we start?"

If a junior nurse feels safe enough to say, "Dr. Smith, I noticed the patient missed his inhaler this morning," that safety culture just saved a life. If they are too scared to speak, the patient risks bronchospasm.

Debriefing: Leadership is also about "closing the loop." After a severe reaction or a difficult clinic, you must lead a "Hot Debrief." This is not an investigation; it is a check-in. "Are we all okay? What went well? What can we fix for tomorrow?" This prevents burnout and builds resilience.

2.3 Quality Management and Accreditation: Beyond the "Tick-Box"

Quality is often mistaken for bureaucracy. In the past, "audit" was something trainees did to fill a portfolio requirement—a quick check of whether 50 patients had their blood pressure recorded. In 2026, we demand more. We demand a culture of safety that is woven into the fabric of the department.

The Philosophy: Audit vs. Improvement

To lead a service, you must distinguish between measuring performance and improving it.

Clinical Audit is the rearview mirror. It looks backward to see if you met a standard. For example, did 100% of patients starting venom immunotherapy receive a consent form? If the answer is 80%, the audit is done. You know the score.

Quality Improvement (QI) is the navigation system. It fixes the route. If only 80% of patients were consented, a QI project asks why and tests a fix.

Shutterstock

Explore

The Engine of Change: The PDSA Cycle The curriculum mandates the use of Plan-Do-Study-Act (PDSA) cycles. This is the scientific method applied to management.

Plan: "We will introduce a digital consent app to improve compliance."

Do: Test it on 10 patients on Tuesday morning.

Study: "Compliance hit 100%, but the app crashed twice."

Act: Fix the bug and roll it out to the whole clinic next week.

In 2026, we expect ACI trainees to lead these projects, not just participate in them. You must demonstrate that your intervention didn't just change a process, but actually improved patient care or service efficiency.

The Gold Standard: Accreditation (IQAS & QPIDS)

In the UK and Ireland, the "badge of honor" for any service is accreditation by the Royal College of Physicians (RCP).

IQAS (Improving Quality in Allergy Services): For allergy-specific units.

QPIDS (Quality in Primary Immunodeficiency Services): For immunology units.

The 2025 Convergence A crucial update for your 2026 exams is understanding the 2025 Standards Revision. In late 2025, IQAS and QPIDS aligned their standards to create a more unified framework. If you are working in a hybrid center (treating both allergy and PID), you now face a streamlined assessment process.

What do these standards look for? They are rigorous.

Facilities: Do you have a dedicated resuscitation trolley in the challenge room? Is the airflow sufficient for sputum induction?

Staffing: Is there a designated lead for pediatric transition? Are clinical nurse specialists empowered to lead their own clinics?

Patient Information: Is your written advice accessible to someone with low literacy or visual impairment?

Learning Through "The Gap Analysis" As a trainee, your most valuable exercise is the Gap Analysis. This is where you take the IQAS/QPIDS standards and walk through your department, identifying where you fall short. It is a humble, eye-opening process. You might realize that while your clinical judgment is excellent, your "clinical governance"—the system that ensures safety—is fragile.

When Things Go Wrong: SUI and RCA

No system is perfect. In 2026, we do not blame individuals for errors; we blame systems.

Serious Untoward Incidents (SUIs): These are major events—for example, a patient receiving the wrong venom dose and suffering anaphylaxis.

Root Cause Analysis (RCA): This is the forensic investigation of the SUI.

Case Study: The Swiss Cheese Model Imagine a patient was given 10x the dose of omalizumab.

Old Way: Blame the nurse.

RCA Way: Why did the nurse draw that amount? Because the vials look identical? (Latent failure). Why was there no double-check? (Process failure). Why was the prescription unclear? (Communication failure).

Your role as a consultant is to lead these RCAs, transforming a disaster into a safety mechanism that prevents recurrence.

2.4 Digital Health and Remote Care Models: The "Hybrid" Immunologist

The 2020 pandemic forced us to adopt digital tools. The years between 2020 and 2025 refined them. Now, in 2026, digital health is not an "add-on"; it is the chassis upon which our service is built.

The New Triage: Remote vs. Face-to-Face

We have moved away from the binary debate of "remote is bad" vs. "remote is good." We now practice Precision Triage.

The "History-First" Model: In many 2026 clinics, the first contact is digital. A video call takes a detailed history. If the history suggests Urticaria, the patient might never need to visit the hospital physically; they can be managed via an app and prescription.

The "Procedure-Only" Slot: Face-to-face slots are precious resources reserved for patients who need physical interaction: skin prick testing, spirometry, or physical examination.

Example:

Patient A (Peanut Allergy): Video consult for history -> Sent for specific IgE blood test locally -> Video review of results. Zero hospital visits.

Patient B (Complex Asthma): Video consult history -> "One-stop shop" visit for CT scan, FeNO, and spirometry on the same day. High-value hospital visit.

The "Virtual Ward": Hospital at Home

One of the most exciting developments in the 2026 curriculum is the operationalization of Virtual Wards for immunology. This concept, pioneered in respiratory medicine, has now reached us.

How it works in 2026: Imagine a patient with Hereditary Angioedema (HAE) or a severe asthma exacerbation.

Instead of keeping them in a hospital bed "just in case," we send them home with a Remote Monitoring Kit.

Connected Devices: A Bluetooth spirometer and pulse oximeter link to a central dashboard at the hospital.

The Safety Net: If their peak flow drops by 15% or their O2 saturation dips, an alarm triggers in the "Virtual Control Room," prompting an immediate video call or ambulance dispatch.

This allows patients to recover in their own beds, reducing hospital-acquired infections and improving mental well-being, while maintaining consultant-level oversight.
Artificial Intelligence: The "Second Opinion"

By 2026, the hype around AI has settled into practical utility. We don't expect AI to replace us, but we expect it to stop us from making mistakes.

1. Predictive Analytics in Food Challenges We now have access to machine learning models that analyze "complex datasets"—combining SpO2, skin prick wheal size, component-resolved diagnostics (Ara h 2), and clinical history—to predict the outcome of a food challenge.

The Benefit: If the AI predicts a 95% chance of reaction, we might skip the dangerous challenge and proceed straight to immunotherapy or avoidance, sparing the patient the trauma of anaphylaxis.

2. Decision Support in Primary Care AI tools are now embedded in GP systems. When a GP types "runny nose" and "wheeze," the AI prompts them to check for atopy before referring. This filters out inappropriate referrals, ensuring that when a patient reaches you, they genuinely need your expertise.

3. The Governance of Data (Generic CiP 5) With great power comes great responsibility. The 2026 curriculum places a massive emphasis on Cybersecurity and Privacy.

You must understand GDPR 2.0 (or the prevailing 2026 equivalent).

You must know how to anonymize data for research.

You must be the guardian of your patient's "Digital Twin"—their accumulated health data.

Conclusion: The Complete Clinician

As we conclude this module, look at the synergy between these two topics.

Quality Management provides the safety rails—ensuring that our processes are robust and our errors are learning opportunities.

Digital Health provides the engine—allowing us to reach patients in their homes, predict their needs using AI, and manage their conditions with unprecedented precision.

Core Laboratory Immunology and Genomics

Part 1: Principles of Diagnostic Testing

1.1 The Physics of Protein Quantification: Nephelometry and Turbidimetry

When we measure immunoglobulins (IgG, IgA, IgM) or complement proteins (C3, C4), we are essentially measuring "cloudiness" in a liquid. However, the method matters.

Turbidimetry works on the principle of occlusion. Imagine you are driving through fog. The fog blocks the light from your headlights. In the lab, we mix the patient's serum with specific antibodies. These antibodies bind to the target protein (antigen), forming immune complexes. These complexes act like the fog. A light source is beamed through the tube, and a detector on the exact opposite side measures how much light was lost.

The Rule: Turbidimetry is generally better for proteins in high concentrations (like total IgG) because there is enough "fog" to measure the blockage accurately.

Nephelometry is different. It relies on light scattering. Instead of looking at the light that passes through, the detector is placed at an angle (usually 70° to 90°) to the light source. It measures the light that bounces off the immune complexes.

The Analogy: Think of dust motes dancing in a sunbeam. You only see them because they scatter the light sideways.

Clinical Application: Nephelometry is more sensitive. It is the gold standard for detecting lower-concentration proteins or early immune complex formation.

2026 Context: Modern analyzers now use "rate" nephelometry. Instead of waiting for the reaction to finish (end-point), the machine measures how fast the cloudiness forms. This creates a kinetic curve that improves accuracy and speed, allowing for higher throughput in busy NHS or private labs.

1.2 The Specific IgE Assay: ELISA and ImmunoCAP

The search for allergy is the search for specific IgE (sIgE). The "RAST" test is a historical relic; do not use this term. The modern standard is the ImmunoCAP (a fluoroenzyme immunoassay).

The Mechanism:

The Sponge: The "CAP" contains a cellulose sponge coated with the allergen (e.g., Peanut Ara h 2). This sponge has a massive surface area, allowing it to catch even tiny amounts of IgE.

The Catch: Patient serum is added. If sIgE is present, it binds to the allergen.

The Signal: We wash away everything else and add an anti-IgE antibody tagged with an enzyme. When a developing solution is added, the enzyme glows (fluorescence). The brightness of the glow is directly proportional to the amount of IgE.

Why it matters: The high capacity of the sponge means we can detect very low levels of sensitization (down to 0.10 kUA/L) without high background noise.

1.3 Autoantibody Screening: Indirect Immunofluorescence (IIF)

Despite the rise of automated bead assays, Indirect Immunofluorescence (IIF) on HEp-2 cells remains the gold standard for screening Anti-Nuclear Antibodies (ANA).

The Process: We take microscope slides coated with human epithelial cells (HEp-2 cells). These cells are huge and have large nuclei, making them perfect display screens. We add patient serum. If autoantibodies are present, they stick to the cell structures. We then add a fluorescent marker.

Pattern Recognition: This is where the art meets science. The pattern of the glow tells you the target.

Homogeneous: The whole nucleus glows. Often associated with anti-dsDNA (Lupus).

Speckled: Polka dots inside the nucleus. Associated with anti-Ro/La (Sjogren's) or anti-Sm.

Centromere: A zipper-like pattern on dividing cells. Classic for Limited Systemic Sclerosis (CREST).

2026 Update: By 2026, manual microscopy is rare. We now rely on Digital AI Microscopy. Algorithms photograph the slides and pre-classify the patterns (e.g., "Probability of Nucleolar Pattern: 98%"). However, your job as an immunologist is to validate the AI. The machine can be fooled by artifacts; the human eye provides the final clinical correlation.

Part 2: Limitations, Interferences, and The "Biological Lie"

A test result is only a number. It becomes a diagnosis only when interpreted correctly. You must be vigilant against laboratory artifacts.

2.1 The Hook Effect (Prozone Phenomenon)

This is a classic trap in nephelometry. It occurs when a patient has an extremely high level of protein (e.g., a massive IgA spike in Myeloma).

The Chemistry: Ideally, you want an equal balance of antigen and antibody to form a lattice structure that scatters light.

The Error: If there is too much patient antigen, the antibodies get swamped. They coat the antigens but cannot link them together to form a lattice. The mixture stays clear.

The Result: The machine reads "Low Signal" and reports a falsely low result.

The Fix: If the clinical picture suggests high disease burden (e.g., a patient with known Myeloma) but the result is normal, ask the lab to dilute the sample. Dilution reduces the antigen excess, allowing the lattice to form, and the "true" high value is revealed.

2.2 Heterophilic Antibodies and HAMA

Some patients have antibodies that stick to animal proteins. These are called Heterophilic antibodies (or HAMA - Human Anti-Mouse Antibodies).

Since many lab assays use mouse antibodies to detect human proteins, these "sticky" patient antibodies can bridge the gap artificially. They create a signal even when the target disease protein is absent.

Example: A patient has a persistently elevated Tryptase or hCG that doesn't fit the symptoms.

The Test: Use a "Blocking Tube" (contains a soup of junk animal protein to soak up the sticky antibodies) or switch to a different assay platform.

2.3 Pre-Analytical Variables: Complement Stability

Complement proteins (C3, C4, and especially the function CH50) are notoriously fragile. They degrade at room temperature.

The Scenario: A GP sends a sample for C3/C4 via standard mail. It sits in a van for 24 hours.

The Consequence: The proteins break down. The lab reports "Low C3/C4." You might misdiagnose Systemic Lupus Erythematosus (SLE) based on a spoiled sample.

Advice to Colleagues: Complement samples must be transported on ice and separated immediately. If the sample wasn't handled right, the result is noise, not data.

2.4 Reference Ranges vs. Clinical Decision Limits

A "Reference Range" is statistical—it usually captures the central 95% of a healthy population. By definition, 5% of healthy people fall outside this range.

The Lesson: Slightly low IgM or borderline low IgG in an asymptomatic person is often a statistical quirk, not a disease.

Clinical Decision Limits are different. These are cut-offs where pathology is likely.

Example: In Tryptase measurement, the reference range might go up to 11.4 ug/L. However, the clinical decision limit for diagnosing Mastocytosis involves a calculated baseline increase (Current > 1.2 x Baseline + 2). You must treat the patient, not the asterisk on the lab report.

Part 3: Cellular Immunology and Flow Cytometry

3.1 Demystifying the Dot Plot

Flow cytometry is the high-speed sorting of cells. Imagine a stream of water so narrow that cells are forced to align in single file. As they pass a laser interrogation point, they scatter light.

The Scattergram: This is your map. It usually has two axes:

Forward Scatter (FSC): X-axis. Measures size. Bigger cells (monocytes) are further right; smaller cells (lymphocytes) are on the left.

Side Scatter (SSC): Y-axis. Measures complexity or "granularity." Granulocytes (neutrophils) are full of granules, so they sit high up. Lymphocytes are smooth, so they sit low.

Gating: "Gating" is simply drawing a circle around the population you want to study. For immune deficiency, we draw a gate around the "Lymphocyte" cloud (small, non-granular). We then ignore everything else (neutrophils, debris).

3.2 Lymphocyte Subsets: T, B, and NK Cells

Once we have gated the lymphocytes, we use fluorochromes (colored tags) attached to antibodies (CD markers) to identify who is who.

CD3: The universal ID card for T-Cells.

CD4: The "Helper" T-cells. Low in HIV and some SCID.

CD8: The "Cytotoxic" T-cells.

CD19 or CD20: The markers for B-Cells (antibody factories). Absent in X-linked Agammaglobulinemia (XLA).

CD16 / CD56: The markers for Natural Killer (NK) cells.

Clinical Patterns:

SCID (Severe Combined Immunodeficiency): You might see a total absence of T-cells (CD3 negative). The scattergram looks empty in the CD3 region.

CVID (Common Variable Immunodeficiency): T-cells might be normal, but B-cells (CD19) could be low or functionally immature (lack of Switched Memory B-cells).

2026 Context: Spectral Cytometry has largely replaced conventional compensation. We now look at the full emission spectrum of a fluorochrome, allowing us to run 20-30 color panels easily. This means we can phenotype naïve, memory, and effector cells in a single tube.

Part 4: Functional Cellular Assays

Counting cells is not enough. We need to know if they work.

4.1 The DHR Test (Neutrophil Oxidative Burst)

Chronic Granulomatous Disease (CGD) is a failure of neutrophils to kill bacteria. They can eat the bacteria (phagocytosis), but they cannot produce the bleach (reactive oxygen species) needed to kill them.

The Assay: We feed the neutrophils a dye called Dihydrorhodamine (DHR).

Healthy Neutrophils: When stimulated, they produce oxygen bursts. This oxidizes the DHR, making it glow bright green (Rhodamine). The histogram shifts to the right (high fluorescence).

CGD Neutrophils: They cannot burst. The DHR stays dark. The histogram stays on the left.

The Genetics in the Graph:

X-Linked CGD (Boys): Usually zero function. A single peak on the far left.

Carrier Mother (X-linked): She has two populations of neutrophils (due to X-inactivation). You will see a "double hump" or bimodal peak—one population works (healthy X), one fails (mutated X).

Autosomal Recessive CGD: The enzyme is partially broken but not gone. You might see a "dim" shift—the whole curve moves slightly right, but not as far as a healthy control.

4.2 Lymphocyte Proliferation Assays

To test T-cell function, we try to make them divide in a test tube.

Mitogens (PHA): These are like a sledgehammer. They stimulate all T-cells regardless of specificity. If cells don't divide to PHA, the T-cells are profoundly broken (e.g., SCID).

Antigens (Tetanus, Candida): This is a memory test. The T-cells should only divide if the patient has been vaccinated or exposed before. It tests the precision of the immune system.

(Note: In a visual guide, this would show peaks halving in brightness as cells divide and split the dye).

4.3 Basophil Activation Test (BAT): The 2026 Frontier

By 2026, the Basophil Activation Test (BAT) has moved from research labs to specialized tertiary networks. It is the ultimate "functional allergy test."

The Problem: Skin tests and specific IgE (ImmunoCAP) only tell you if IgE is present (sensitization). They do not tell you if the cells will actually explode and cause anaphylaxis (clinical allergy).

The Solution: We take live patient blood (containing basophils). We add the allergen (e.g., Amoxicillin or Peanut) in the test tube.

The Marker: If the basophil recognizes the allergen and activates, it pushes a hidden protein to its surface: CD63 or CD203c.

The Measurement: We use flow cytometry to count how many basophils are expressing CD63.

Clinical Utility: BAT is crucial for "equivocal" cases.

Example: A patient has a borderline peanut skin test but a terrifying history. A BAT challenge is safer than feeding them a peanut. If the BAT is negative, we can often proceed to oral food challenge with confidence.

Drug Allergy: BAT is revolutionizing the diagnosis of immediate reactions to muscle relaxants and antibiotics where skin testing is often irritating or unreliable.

Conclusion

Diagnostic immunology is a discipline of nuance. As a specialist in 2026, you are the guardian of interpretation. The technology—from rapid nephelometry to spectral flow cytometry—provides the data points. But it is your understanding of the physics, the limitations, and the cellular biology that converts that data into a diagnosis.

3.3 Molecular Allergology: Component Resolved Diagnostics (CRD)

The Philosophy of Precision: Extracts vs. Components

To understand Component Resolved Diagnostics (CRD), you must first understand the limitations of the past. Whole allergen extracts—whether used in SPT or specific IgE (sIgE) blood tests—are crude biological mixtures. A peanut extract contains dangerous storage proteins, harmless pollen-related proteins, and confusing carbohydrate structures all mixed together.

Testing with an extract is like trying to identify a criminal by looking at a crowd of people. You might see the crowd (positive test), but you don't know if the criminal (the dangerous allergen) is actually there.

CRD allows us to pick individuals out of the crowd. We can test for specific proteins to answer three critical questions:

Is the risk systemic (anaphylaxis) or local (oral symptoms)?

Is this a primary sensitization or a cross-reaction?

Is the positive test a technical artifact (CCD)?

The Paradigm of Peanut Allergy: Ara h 2 vs. Ara h 8

Peanut allergy remains the best model for teaching CRD because the clinical stakes are so high. In 2026, we no longer rely solely on "Peanut IgE." We look at the profile.
1. The Storage Proteins: The "Danger" Signals (Ara h 2, 6)

Ara h 2 (2S Albumin): This is the villain of the story. Ara h 2 is a seed storage protein designed by nature to survive desiccation and germination. Chemically, it is tightly wound with disulfide bridges, making it incredibly stable against heat and digestion.

Clinical Reality: When a patient eats a roasted peanut, the Ara h 2 survives the roasting pan and the stomach acid, arriving intact at the intestinal mast cells to trigger a massive release of histamine.

2026 Guideline: If a child has high sIgE to Ara h 2 (typically >0.35 kU/L, though 2026 cutoffs have become more nuanced based on age), the likelihood of anaphylaxis is >95%. We do not challenge these patients. They need an adrenaline autoinjector.

Ara h 6: Often travels with Ara h 2. It is functionally similar. If Ara h 2 is positive, Ara h 6 is almost always positive.

2. The PR-10 Proteins: The "Pollen" Ghosts (Ara h 8)

Ara h 8: This protein is a structural homolog of Bet v 1, the major birch pollen allergen. It is widespread in the plant kingdom.

Stability: Unlike Ara h 2, Ara h 8 is fragile. It falls apart when heated or exposed to pepsin in the stomach.

Clinical Reality: A patient sensitized to birch pollen (hay fever) will have IgE that cross-reacts with Ara h 8. When they do a whole peanut test, it comes back positive. However, when they eat a peanut, the Ara h 8 is destroyed by their stomach acid before it can cause a systemic reaction. They might feel a tingle in the mouth (Oral Allergy Syndrome), but they will not go into shock.

2026 Guideline: A patient who is Ara h 8 positive but Ara h 2 negative is a prime candidate for an Oral Food Challenge (OFC) or, in many low-risk cases, home introduction. We can often liberate these patients from the burden of avoidance.

3. The Lipid Transfer Proteins (Ara h 9)

Ara h 9: This fits in the middle. It is an LTP, common in the Mediterranean region (associated with peach allergy, Pru p 3). It is stable enough to cause systemic reactions but often requires a cofactor (exercise, NSAIDs) to trigger anaphylaxis.

Beyond the Peanut: Hazelnut, Venom, and Latex

Once you master the peanut model, you can apply the same logic to other allergens. The names change, but the protein families—and the risks—remain the same.

Hazelnut: A Tale of Two Geographies

In Northern Europe (and parts of North America), hazelnut allergy is usually mild. In the Mediterranean, it is severe. CRD explains why.

The "North" Profile (Cor a 1): This is a PR-10 protein, a cousin of the birch pollen allergen. Just like Ara h 8, it causes mild oral symptoms. A child with high Cor a 1 and low Cor a 9/14 can usually eat Nutella (processed/heated hazelnut) safely.

The "South" Profile (Cor a 9, Cor a 14): These are the storage proteins (11S globulin and 2S albumin). They are heat-stable and dangerous.

Cor a 14: In 2026, this is considered the superior marker for pediatric systemic risk. If Cor a 14 is elevated, the risk of anaphylaxis is high, regardless of the geographic location.

Venom Allergy: solving the "Double Positive"

Hymenoptera (insect sting) allergy is a high-stakes field. A patient stung by a "flying insect" arrives with anaphylaxis. The whole venom test is positive for both Honeybee and Wasp (Yellow Jacket). Are they unlucky enough to be allergic to both? Or is it cross-reactivity?

The Problem: Both bee and wasp venoms contain Hyaluronidases (Api m 2 and Ves v 2). These enzymes are highly cross-reactive due to their sugar structures (CCDs). A patient allergic to bees might test positive for wasp because of these shared sugars.

The Solution (CRD): We test for the species-specific marker components.

Honeybee: Api m 1 (Phospholipase A2). This is the unique signature of the bee.

Wasp (Vespula): Ves v 1 (Phospholipase A1) and Ves v 5 (Antigen 5).

2026 Strategy: If a patient is Api m 1 positive and Ves v 5 negative, they are bee allergic. The wasp positivity was a ghost. This distinction is vital because Venom Immunotherapy (VIT) is specific; giving a wasp vaccine to a bee-allergic patient is a 5-year, expensive mistake.

Latex: The fading epidemic

Latex allergy has declined due to glove manufacturing changes, but it persists in spina bifida patients and healthcare workers.

Hev b 1, 3, 5, 6.01: These are the markers of true latex allergy associated with glove use and surgical anaphylaxis.

Hev b 8 (Profilin): This is the confuser. Profilins are in grass, trees, and weeds. A patient with grass allergy may test positive for Latex Hev b 8 but can wear latex gloves safely. Differentiating Hev b 6 from Hev b 8 prevents unnecessary avoidance in the operating theatre.

The CCD Trap: Cross-Reactive Carbohydrate Determinants

If there is one concept that trips up trainees (and experienced consultants), it is the CCD.

What is a CCD? Plants and insects decorate their proteins with specific sugar chains (N-glycans). These sugars often contain a Core α-1,3-fucose or a β-1,2-xylose. Here is the catch: Mammals (humans) do not make these specific sugar patterns.

The Immune Response: Because these sugars look "foreign," the human immune system often makes IgE antibodies against them.

The Paradox: These anti-CCD IgE antibodies bind avidly in the test tube, causing bright positive results on ImmunoCAP or ISAC. However, they possess low biological affinity in the body. They can grab the allergen, but they cannot cross-link the high-affinity IgE receptors on the mast cell tightly enough to trigger degranulation.

The Result: A "False Positive." The patient has high IgE but no symptoms.

Common Culprits:

Venom: As mentioned, hyaluronidases are rich in CCDs.

Plant Foods: Soy, peanut, and tomato extracts are often CCD-rich.

The 2026 Solution: In modern assays (like the ALEX2/3 macroarray), a CCD Blocker is automatically added. This blocker is a solution of CCDs (often from bromelain) that soaks up the patient's anti-CCD IgE before it can bind to the test chip. This "cleans" the serum, leaving only the

protein-specific IgE to be measured. If you see a raw result with high sensitization to everything (tomato, grass, bee, soy, latex) but the patient is asymptomatic, suspect CCDs.
Technology in 2026: Singleplex vs. Multiplex

Trainees must understand the cost-benefit analysis of the tools at their disposal.
1. Singleplex Assays (e.g., ImmunoCAP)

What it is: Testing one allergen at a time.

Pros: Highly quantitative, the "Gold Standard" for defining cut-offs (e.g., Ara h 2 > 0.35).

Cons: Expensive if you order too many. Requires more serum volume.

Use Case: The patient has a clear history of peanut reaction. You just need to confirm Ara h 2 to decide on an autoinjector.

2. Multiplex Arrays (ISAC, ALEX)

What it is: A biochip containing hundreds (approx. 300 in 2026) of allergen components.

Pros: "Broadcasting." You get the whole picture—pollens, foods, mites, venoms—in one shot. Excellent for the "pollen-food syndrome" patient who reacts to ten different fruits. It automatically sorts out the CCDs and cross-reactions.

Cons: Semi-quantitative. You get "ISU" or "kU/L" but they don't always align perfectly with Singleplex.

Use Case: The patient with "idiopathic" anaphylaxis, or complex eczema with unclear triggers. It helps build a "molecular map" of the patient's sensitization profile.

Section 3.3 Summary: Risk Stratification

The ultimate goal of CRD is Risk Stratification.

Low Risk (OAS/Local): Sensitized to PR-10 (Ara h 8, Cor a 1) or Profilin (Hev b 8).

Management: Likely no EpiPen needed. Can often tolerate processed forms.

High Risk (Systemic/Anaphylaxis): Sensitized to Storage Proteins (Ara h 2, Cor a 14, Ana o 3).

Management: Strict avoidance. Adrenaline autoinjector mandatory.

The "Grey Zone": Lipid Transfer Proteins (Ara h 9, Pru p 3).

Management: Case-by-case. Assess co-factors.

By mastering this module, you spare the PR-10 sensitized child from the social stigma of a "nut free" table, and you protect the Storage Protein sensitized child from a life-threatening error.

3.4 Genomics in Clinical Practice

The Genomic Revolution in Immunology

By 2026, Genomic Medicine is no longer a niche interest for academic researchers; it is the backbone of diagnosing Inborn Errors of Immunity (IEI). We have identified over 550 monogenic causes of immune dysregulation. The old strategy of "phenotyping" (counting

T-cells and measuring immunoglobulins) is now just the screening step. The diagnosis is genetic.

This module aligns with the "Future of Medicine" curriculum. As an ACI physician, you do not need to be a geneticist, but you must be a competent "consumer" of genetic data.

The Hierarchy of Testing

When you suspect a genetic immune disorder (e.g., a child with recurrent abscesses or an adult with Common Variable Immunodeficiency - CVID), you must choose the right tool. In 2026, we utilize a tiered approach, often guided by the National Genomic Test Directory.

1. Targeted Gene Panels

The "Sniper Rifle."

Method: Next-Generation Sequencing (NGS) of a specific list of genes known to cause a specific phenotype.

Example: The "Agammaglobulinemia Panel" looks at BTK, BLNK, μ-heavy chain, etc.

Pros: Deep coverage (reads the gene hundreds of times to ensure accuracy). Fewer "Incidental Findings." Faster turnaround.

Cons: If the patient has a novel gene mutation not on the list, you will miss it.

2. Whole Exome Sequencing (WES)

The "Dragnet."

Method: Sequencing the protein-coding regions (exons) of all ~20,000 genes. This represents only 1-2% of the genome, but it houses ~85% of known disease-causing mutations.

Pros: Good for heterogeneous disorders like CVID or SCID where hundreds of different genes could be the culprit.

Cons: Misses mutations in "introns" (the spacers between code) or complex structural changes.

3. Whole Genome Sequencing (WGS)

The "Satellite Surveillance."

Method: Sequencing everything. Coding, non-coding, regulatory regions.

Status in 2026: WGS is becoming the standard of care for complex IEI.

Why? It detects Structural Variants (SVs) and Copy Number Variants (CNVs) (large deletions or duplications) that WES misses. It also covers deep intronic variants that affect splicing.

The Test Directory: In national health systems (like the NHS or equivalent US insurance models), WGS is now "Green lit" for primary immune deficiencies that evade panel diagnosis.

Interpreting the Report: The Language of Variants

Receiving a genetic report can be daunting. You will not see a simple "Positive/Negative." You will see variants classified according to ACMG (American College of Medical Genetics) criteria.

You must memorize this hierarchy:

Pathogenic (Class 5): >99% certainty it causes disease. This is a diagnosis.

Likely Pathogenic (Class 4): >90% certainty. Usually treated as a diagnosis in clinical practice.

Variant of Uncertain Significance (VUS - Class 3): The "Grey Zone." Probability 10-90%. DO NOT act on this alone.

Likely Benign (Class 2): Harmless.

Benign (Class 1): Harmless.

The VUS Dilemma

The VUS is the bane of the immunologist's existence. You find a mutation in STAT3 in a patient with eczema. Is it the cause (Job's Syndrome)? Or is it just a random genetic typo?

Rule of Thumb: Never use a VUS to justify a bone marrow transplant or irreversible therapy without further proof.

Segregation Analysis: Solving the Puzzle

How do we turn a VUS into a Pathogenic variant? We use Segregation Analysis. This involves testing the parents (and sometimes siblings).

Scenario: You find a heterozygous VUS in STAT1 (Associated with dominant GOF mutations) in a sick child.

Test the Parents:

Result A: The healthy father has the same mutation.

Conclusion: The variant is likely benign (or penetrance is very low). It is unlikely to be the cause of the child's severe disease.

Result B: Neither parent has the mutation. The child has a de novo (new) mutation.

Conclusion: This is strong evidence for pathogenicity. Nature rarely makes de novo errors in conserved genes without consequence. The VUS can often be reclassified to "Likely Pathogenic."

Trio WGS: In 2026, we often sequence the Child + Mother + Father simultaneously (Trio Analysis) to automate this filtering process.
Ethical Considerations and Counseling (Generic CiP 2)

Genomics carries a weight that other tests do not. It affects the whole family.
1. Pre-test Counseling

Before you order WGS, you must consent the patient. This is not just a formality. You must discuss:

The chance of no answer: "We might not find the cause."

The VUS risk: "We might find a change we don't understand, which can be anxiety-provoking."

Incidental Findings: "We might accidentally find a gene for Breast Cancer (BRCA) or Huntington's. Do you want to know?" (The "Right not to know").

2. The Implications for Family

A diagnosis of X-linked Agammaglobulinemia (XLA) in a boy implies his mother is a carrier. This impacts her sisters, her future children, and the wider family tree.

The 2026 Standard: You must have a clear pathway for Cascade Screening—offering testing to at-risk relatives once the proband (index patient) is diagnosed.

3. Insurance and Employment

While many regions have laws against genetic discrimination (like GINA in the US), patients often fear that a genetic diagnosis will make them uninsurable for life insurance. As an ACI physician, you must provide honest, up-to-date advice on these risks.

Anaphylaxis and Acute Emergencies

4.1 Pathophysiology and Diagnosis of Anaphylaxis

The Engine Room: Mechanisms of Shock

To manage anaphylaxis effectively, you must visualize what is happening at the cellular level. When a patient crashes, it is rarely chaos; it is a highly orchestrated cascade of immune errors.

1. IgE-Mediated Anaphylaxis (The Classic Pathway) This is the mechanism most familiar to us. It is the "lock and key" model. A specific allergen (food, venom, drug) cross-links specific IgE antibodies bound to the high-affinity receptor, FcεRI, on the surface of mast cells and basophils.

Think of the mast cell as a loaded mine. The cross-linking of IgE is the pressure plate. Once triggered, the cell degranulates explosively.

Immediate Phase: Within seconds, pre-formed granules serve up a cocktail of histamine, tryptase, and heparin.

Late Phase: Minutes to hours later, the cell machinery synthesizes new lipid mediators like Platelet-Activating Factor (PAF), prostaglandins (PGD2), and leukotrienes (LTC4).

2. Non-IgE Mediated Mechanisms (The New Frontier) Historically, we called these "anaphylactoid" reactions. In 2026, we have discarded that term. It was vague and unhelpful. We now refer to these as non-immunologic anaphylaxis or direct mast cell activation.

The breakthrough here is the MRGPRX2 receptor. For decades, we knew that drugs like morphine, vancomycin, and certain neuromuscular blockers (like atracurium) could cause shock without a prior allergy. We now know why. These drugs bind directly to the MRGPRX2 receptor on the mast cell surface, bypassing IgE entirely. This explains why a patient can react to a drug they have never seen before.

The "Cytokine Storm" and Phenotype Why do patients die? It is not usually the swelling; it is the vascular permeability.

Histamine drives the itch and the hives.

Bradykinin and PAF destroy the integrity of the vascular endothelium. Fluid leaks out of the blood vessels and into the tissues at a terrifying rate—up to 35% of the intravascular volume can shift into the extravascular space within 10 minutes. The heart is pumping against an empty tank (distributive shock).

Diagnosis: The Clinical Eye

The diagnosis of anaphylaxis is clinical. You cannot wait for a blood test. In 2026, we follow the streamlined World Allergy Organization (WAO) criteria. The focus has shifted away from skin signs.

The "Silent" Anaphylaxis (A Fatal Pitfall) Here is a critical clinical pearl: 20% of fatal anaphylaxis cases have no skin signs. If you wait for urticaria (hives) or angioedema (swelling), you will miss the window to save the patient. This is particularly true in:

Rapid-onset insect venom cases.

Perioperative cases (where the patient is covered in drapes).

Fatal food reactions, where respiratory arrest often precedes skin changes.

Diagnostic Criteria (Simplified) Anaphylaxis is highly likely if ANY ONE of the following occurs:

Acute onset (minutes to hours) involving skin/mucosa AND at least one of:

Respiratory compromise (wheeze, stridor).

Reduced Blood Pressure (collapse, incontinence).

Acute onset of hypotension or bronchospasm or laryngeal involvement after exposure to a known or highly probable allergen (even without skin signs).

Retrospective Confirmation: Serum Tryptase While you treat based on clinical suspicion, you confirm based on tryptase. Tryptase is an enzyme stored almost exclusively in mast cells.

Acute Sample: Take this 1–2 hours after the start of symptoms. This catches the peak.

Baseline Sample: Take this 24 hours later (or weeks later in clinic).

The 2026 Formula: A significant rise is defined as:
$\text{Acute Tryptase} > (1.2 \times \text{Baseline Tryptase}) + 2\ \text{ng/mL}$

If the acute level meets this threshold, a mast cell event has occurred.

Differential Diagnosis: The Mimics

Not every collapse is anaphylaxis. We must distinguish the signal from the noise.

Panic Attacks: These are the most common mimic. Patients hyperventilate. They may feel "throat tightness" (globus hystericus) but they do not have stridor. Crucially, panic attacks usually cause hypertension and tachycardia (unless there is a vaso-vagal faint), whereas anaphylaxis causes hypotension.

Scombroid Poisoning: Often confused with fish allergy. This is caused by eating spoiled fish (tuna, mackerel) rich in histidine, which bacteria convert to histamine. The patient ingests pure histamine. They get flushed, have a headache, and may wheeze. It looks like anaphylaxis, but the tryptase will be normal because their own mast cells didn't degranulate.

Vocal Cord Dysfunction (VCD): This presents as sudden "choking" or throat closure. It is terrifying for the patient. However, upon auscultation, the stridor is inspiratory and high-pitched, localized to the throat, often with good oxygen saturation. Adrenaline does not help VCD.

Pheochromocytoma/Carcinoid: Rare tumors that dump mediators (catecholamines or serotonin) into the blood. These cause flushing and shock but usually follow a chronic, episodic pattern.

4.2 Acute Management and Refractory Cases

Immediate Management: Adrenaline is Non-Negotiable

There is no absolute contraindication to adrenaline in a life-threatening crisis. None. Antihistamines (chlorphenamine) and steroids (hydrocortisone) are second-line. They do not save lives in the first 10 minutes. They treat the itch and potentially dampen the late-phase reaction, but they do not reverse shock.

The Route: Intramuscular (IM) Anterolateral Thigh Why the thigh? We inject into the vastus lateralis because it is a massive, highly vascularized muscle. In a patient with shutting-down periphery (shock), blood flow to the skin and subcutaneous fat is clamped off. If you inject adrenaline subcutaneously (like insulin), it will sit there, unabsorbed, while the patient deteriorates. The muscle pump ensures rapid systemic delivery.

Dosing (The 1:1000 Rule)

Adults: 0.5 mg (0.5 mL of 1:1000 solution).

Children: 0.01 mg/kg (up to 0.3 mg or 0.5 mg depending on age/weight).

Posture is Critical Never, ever stand an anaphylactic patient up. When the blood vessels dilate, the "tank" is bigger. If you stand the patient up, gravity drains the remaining blood volume away from the brain and heart. This can cause "Empty Ventricle Syndrome" and immediate cardiac arrest. Keep them supine with legs raised. If they are struggling to breathe, sit them up slightly, but keep the legs extended.

Refractory Anaphylaxis

What happens when the adrenaline doesn't work? Refractory anaphylaxis is defined as a reaction that requires ongoing treatment despite two appropriate IM doses of adrenaline.

Step 1: Fluid Resuscitation The vascular leak is massive. You must refill the tank.

Use large-bore IV access (grey or orange cannula).

Give a rapid bolus of crystalloid (Hartmann's or Saline): 20 mL/kg. In an adult, this is often 1–2 liters stat.

Step 2: Intravenous Adrenaline Infusion If IM fails, we move to IV.

Warning: IV adrenaline is dangerous. It can cause hypertensive crisis and arrhythmias if given as a bolus to a patient with a pulse.

The Protocol: We typically use a dilute solution.

Mix 1 mg adrenaline in 100 mL saline (making a 10 mcg/mL solution).

Start infusion at 0.5–1 mL/kg/hour and titrate to blood pressure.

This requires continuous ECG monitoring.

Step 3: The Beta-Blocked Patient Patients on beta-blockers (e.g., bisoprolol, atenolol) have a "blocked" receptor site. Adrenaline (an alpha and beta agonist) may struggle to activate the heart.

The Antidote: Glucagon.

Glucagon activates the heart via a non-adrenergic pathway (increasing cAMP). It bypasses the beta-blocker blockade.

Dose: 1–5 mg IV bolus over 5 minutes, followed by an infusion if necessary. Note: It often makes the patient vomit, so protect the airway.

Perioperative Anaphylaxis (2026 Context)

Managing anaphylaxis in the operating theater is a unique challenge. The patient cannot speak. They cannot tell you "my throat is tight" or "I feel doom."

The NAP6 Legacy and Beyond

The 6th National Audit Project (NAP6) in the UK remains the gold standard study for perioperative anaphylaxis, and its lessons are integral to 2026 practice.

Presentation in the Anaesthetized Patient

Hypotension: Present in 100% of severe cases. If the BP drops suddenly after induction, assume anaphylaxis until proven otherwise.

Bronchospasm: Common, especially in asthmatics.

Skin signs: Often absent or covered by surgical drapes. Do not rely on them.

The Common Culprits

Antibiotics: Specifically Teicoplanin and Co-amoxiclav. In 2026, antibiotic sensitization is the leading cause.

Neuromuscular Blocking Agents (NMBAs):

Suxamethonium is a high-risk trigger for IgE-mediated reactions.

Atracurium often causes histamine release via the MRGPRX2 receptor (non-IgE), presenting as hypotension without true allergy.

Rocuronium: A common cause of IgE-mediated anaphylaxis.

Chlorhexidine: The antiseptic used to clean the skin or coat central lines. It is an insidious, often delayed trigger.

Patent Blue Dye: Used in breast surgery sentinel node biopsy. It causes a delayed reaction (30-60 mins) and interferes with pulse oximetry readings (blue blood looks deoxygenated).

Management in Theatre

Stop the Trigger: If you are infusing an antibiotic, stop it. If you are inducing, pause surgery.

Airway: Intubate immediately if not already done. Anaphylactic edema can close the glottis in seconds.

Specific Investigations:

Mast Cell Tryptase: Take immediately, then at 2 hours, then at 24 hours.

Referral: All perioperative cases must be referred to a specialist drug allergy clinic. We will test for the specific agents using skin prick testing and specific IgE.

4.3 Long-Term Management and Adrenaline Autoinjectors (AAIs)

Surviving an anaphylactic event is a traumatic physiological and psychological experience. Effective long-term management relies on three pillars: Device Competency, Personalized Action Plans, and Psychosocial Support.

The Diversification of Delivery Devices

For decades, the intramuscular (IM) "stab" was the only option for patients. Today, the landscape is broader. As a clinician in 2026, you must be competent in prescribing and teaching the full range of licensed devices.

1. Traditional Autoinjectors (The "Needle" Class)

Despite innovation, traditional AAIs remain a staple for many patients, particularly those with specific physiological profiles or severe hypotension histories where IM delivery is preferred.

EpiPen & EpiPen Jr: The veteran device. It uses a spring-loaded needle activated by pressure against the thigh.

Jext: Similar mechanism to EpiPen but with a different locking safety cap.

Anapen: Distinguishable by its thumb-plunger activation mechanism, which some patients with dexterity issues find easier to control than the "swing and jab" motion.

Clinical Example: A construction worker with callous, thick skin on their hands might struggle with the fine motor skills needed to remove small safety caps during a reaction. In this case, you might prescribe a device with a more robust gripping mechanism or the new needle-free options.

2. The Needle-Free Revolution: Mucosal Epinephrine

The approval of neffy (nasal epinephrine) in the EU and UK (2025) marked a paradigm shift. This device delivers epinephrine via the nasal mucosa, bypassing the need for an injection.

Mechanism: It uses an absorption enhancer to allow large epinephrine molecules to cross the nasal membrane rapidly.

Indication: It is currently licensed for patients >30kg.

Pros: It eliminates "needle phobia," a major barrier to use. Studies show that patients (and bystanders) are far more likely to administer a nasal spray early in a reaction than they are to use a needle.

Cons: It requires a clear nasal passage. While it works even with nasal congestion, significant anatomical blockages (like polyps) might be a relative contraindication, though 2026 data suggests high efficacy even in rhinitis.

Clinical Example: Consider a teenager who refuses to carry their AAI to school because they are terrified of needles and embarrassed by the bulky device. Switching them to a nasal device, which looks like a common allergy spray, can increase compliance from 0% to 100%.

Personalized Anaphylaxis Action Plans (AAPs)

A generic plan is a useless plan. In 2026, we emphasize "context-aware" action plans. You must tailor the plan to the patient's specific environment.

Schools: The plan must be "teacher-proof." It needs simple graphics (QR codes linking to video tutorials are now standard on 2026 plans) and clear instructions on who holds the device.

Travel: For patients flying internationally, the plan acts as a "medical passport" to allow liquid medication through security. It must also include the generic names of medication, as brand names like "EpiPen" are not used globally.

The "Vigilance Burden": Patients often suffer from decision fatigue. Your plan should simplify their choices. Instead of "If you feel X, maybe do Y," use binary language: "If breathing is difficult -> USE DEVICE."

Psychosocial Impact: Beyond the Biology

Anaphylaxis carries a heavy mental load. We now recognize Post-Anaphylaxis Distress Syndrome (PADS) as a real clinical entity.

Needle Phobia: This is not just "disliking shots." It is a visceral, paralyzing fear that causes patients to delay life-saving treatment. The introduction of nasal epinephrine has been a major breakthrough here, but cognitive behavioral therapy (CBT) referrals are still necessary for severe cases.

Vigilance Fatigue: Patients get tired of reading every label, every time. This leads to risky behaviors, especially in adolescents.

Support for Carers (CiP 5): Parents of allergic children often suffer higher anxiety than the patients themselves. Teaching a parent how to use a device is not a one-time event. Skills decay happens within 3-6 months. You must schedule "refresher" training at every clinic visit.

4.4 Idiopathic Anaphylaxis and Mast Cell Disorders

When a patient presents with anaphylaxis and standard allergy tests (skin prick, specific IgE) are negative, we enter the realm of complex investigations. Do not jump to the

"Idiopathic" label too quickly. "Idiopathic" simply means "we haven't found the cause yet."
The "Hidden" Allergens (Occult Triggers)

Before diagnosing Idiopathic Anaphylaxis (IA), you must rule out these three sophisticated masqueraders.
1. Alpha-gal Syndrome (Red Meat Allergy)

This is a delayed allergy caused by a sugar molecule (galactose-alpha-1,3-galactose) found in mammalian meat (beef, pork, lamb), but not in humans, fish, or birds.

The Vector: Sensitization occurs via tick bites (e.g., Ixodes ricinus in Europe/UK, Amblyomma americanum in the US). The tick saliva primes the immune system against the sugar.

The Trap: Unlike a peanut allergy which reacts in minutes, Alpha-gal reactions occur 3 to 6 hours after eating. A patient might eat a steak for dinner, go to sleep, and wake up in anaphylaxis at 2:00 AM.

Diagnosis: Specific IgE to Alpha-gal.

Clinical Example: A patient presents with recurrent "midnight anaphylaxis." They have no history of food allergy. A forensic history reveals they enjoy weekend hiking (tick exposure) and often eat burgers for dinner. This is classic Alpha-gal.

2. Omega-5-Gliadin (Wheat-Dependent Exercise-Induced Anaphylaxis)

This is the most common cause of "unexplained" adult anaphylaxis. The patient is not allergic to wheat in a traditional sense. They can eat bread and sit on the couch safely. They can go for a run safely. But if they eat bread AND go for a run within 4 hours, they react.

Mechanism: Exercise increases gut permeability, allowing the large Omega-5-gliadin protein to enter the bloodstream and trigger mast cells.

Cofactors: It's not just exercise. Alcohol, NSAIDs (like ibuprofen), and menstruation can also act as "keys" that unlock the reaction.

Diagnosis: Specific IgE to Omega-5-gliadin (rTri a 19).

3. Lipid Transfer Proteins (LTPs)

LTPs are pan-allergens found in the skins of many fruits and vegetables (peaches, apples, tomatoes). They are heat-stable (cooking doesn't destroy them) and digestion-resistant. In Southern Europe, this is a dominant cause of "idiopathic" reactions.

Mast Cell Disorders: When the Cell is the Problem

If you have ruled out all external triggers, you must look inside. Is the patient's immune system hyper-reactive?

The Diagnostic Algorithm

We differentiate between Systemic Mastocytosis (SM) (a neoplastic disease where mast cells multiply abnormally) and Mast Cell Activation Syndrome (MCAS) (where mast cells are normal in number but hyper-functional).

Baseline Tryptase: Every patient with unexplained anaphylaxis needs a baseline serum tryptase test (taken 24+ hours after a reaction).

Normal is < 11.4 ng/mL.

Levels > 20 ng/mL are a "Minor Criterion" for Systemic Mastocytosis.

The "20% + 2" Rule: To confirm mast cell activation during a reaction, you compare the acute tryptase (taken 1-4 hours after symptoms) to the baseline.

Formula: Acute Level > (1.2 × Baseline) + 2.

Example: Baseline is 5 ng/mL. The activation threshold is (1.2 × 5) + 2 = 8 ng/mL. If the patient's acute level is 10 ng/mL, activation is confirmed.

Systemic Mastocytosis (SM)

In 2026, the management of SM has been revolutionized by precision medicine.

The Mutation: Over 90% of SM patients have the KIT D816V mutation. This is a "stuck gas pedal" mutation that keeps mast cells turned on.

Diagnosis: If tryptase is elevated, we proceed to a highly sensitive PCR blood test for KIT D816V. If positive, a bone marrow biopsy follows to look for aberrant mast cells (CD25+).

Treatment (The 2026 Update): We now use Tyrosine Kinase Inhibitors (TKIs) like Avapritinib. Unlike older drugs, Avapritinib specifically targets the KIT D816V mutation. It essentially "cuts the fuel line" to the rogue mast cells. It is effective even in Indolent Systemic Mastocytosis (ISM) for symptom control when antihistamines fail.

Clinical Example: A patient has suffered monthly anaphylactic shock for 10 years, living in fear. Diagnosis reveals Systemic Mastocytosis.

Respiratory Allergy: Asthma and Rhinitis

5.1 Allergic Rhinitis and Comorbidities

The Burden of Disease

Respiratory allergy is likely the most common condition you will encounter in your clinic. While it is rarely fatal, its impact on quality of life—sleep, cognitive function, and productivity—is profound. As of 2026, the economic burden of untreated rhinitis rivals that of diabetes.

Classification: Beyond the Sneeze

We utilize the ARIA (Allergic Rhinitis and its Impact on Asthma) guidelines as our roadmap. The old classification of "seasonal" versus "perennial" is largely obsolete because many patients are polysensitized (allergic to multiple things) and have symptoms year-round.

Instead, ARIA classifies rhinitis based on duration (Intermittent vs. Persistent) and severity (Mild vs. Moderate-Severe).

Intermittent: Symptoms present <4 days a week or <4 consecutive weeks.

Persistent: Symptoms present >4 days a week and >4 consecutive weeks.

Differential Diagnosis: The "Non-Allergic" Pitfall Not every runny nose is allergic. One of your primary skills is differentiating Allergic Rhinitis (AR) from Non-Allergic Rhinitis (NAR).

Vasomotor Rhinitis: This is the "over-sensitive" nose. Triggers aren't allergens like pollen, but irritants: cold air, strong perfumes, smoke, or pollution. The neural reflex arc is hyperactive.

Gustatory Rhinitis: The classic "runny nose while eating," particularly with spicy foods.

Hormonal Rhinitis: Often seen in pregnancy ("pregnancy rhinitis") or with hypothyroidism.

The Mystery of Local Allergic Rhinitis (LAR) For years, patients with classic allergy symptoms but negative skin prick tests and negative blood IgE were told they had "non-allergic rhinitis." We now know many of them have Local Allergic Rhinitis (LAR).

In LAR, the systemic immune system is quiet, but the local nasal mucosa is producing specific IgE antibodies. It is a localized rebellion. Diagnosis often requires a Nasal Allergen Challenge (NAC), where you provoke the nose with the allergen and monitor for a drop in airflow or symptom spikes.
The United Airway Theory

"One Airway, One Disease."

This is the central dogma of modern allergy practice. The upper airway (nose/sinuses) and lower airway (lungs/bronchi) are lined by the same respiratory epithelium. They are connected physically and immunologically.

The Link: If you dump inflammatory cytokines in the nose (e.g., during ragweed season), those cytokines enter the systemic circulation and upregulate inflammation in the lungs.

Clinical Implication: You cannot successfully manage difficult asthma if you ignore the patient's dripping nose. Treating the rhinitis often improves asthma control.

Comorbidities: The Difficult Cases

1. Chronic Rhinosinusitis with Nasal Polyps (CRSwNP) This is a severe, debilitating T2-high inflammatory condition. Patients often present with anosmia (loss of smell) and nasal obstruction. The polyps are like "peeled grapes"—pale, insensitive masses obstructing the airway. By 2026, our management has shifted heavily toward biologics (anti-IL-4/IL-13 or anti-IgE) for recurrent cases, sparing patients from repeated, mutilating surgeries.

2. Aspirin-Exacerbated Respiratory Disease (AERD) Also known as Samter's Triad, this is a fascinating and dangerous phenotype. It consists of three pillars:

Asthma.

CRSwNP (Nasal Polyps).

Hypersensitivity to Aspirin/NSAIDs.

The Mechanism (The COX-1 Crisis): Imagine a factory line producing inflammatory chemicals.

Normally, the enzyme COX-1 helps produce Prostaglandin E2 (PGE2). PGE2 acts as a "brake" on inflammation.

In AERD patients, taking aspirin blocks COX-1.

This removes the PGE2 "brake."

Simultaneously, the metabolic pathway shifts aggressively toward the Lipoxygenase pathway.

Result: A massive overproduction of Cysteinyl Leukotrienes (CysLTs). These are potent constrictors of the airway.

The patient takes an aspirin for a headache and, within 30 minutes, experiences a violent asthma attack and nasal congestion.
Practical Skills: The Eyes of the ACI Physician

Anterior Rhinoscopy This is your basic screening tool. Using a Thudicum speculum or otoscope, you look for:

Pale, boggy turbinates: Suggests Allergic Rhinitis.

Red, inflamed mucosa: Suggests infection or rhinitis medicamentosa (addiction to nasal decongestant sprays).

Septal deviation: A mechanical blockage.

Nasendoscopy This is the gold standard. A flexible fiberoptic scope is passed into the nasal cavity. You must learn to interpret:

The Osteomeatal Complex (OMC): The drainage pathway for the sinuses. If this is blocked by polyps or edema, sinusitis is inevitable.

Adenoidal Hypertrophy: Especially in younger adults or children, which can mimic allergic congestion.

5.2 Asthma Phenotypes and Endotypes

The Death of "Generic" Asthma

In the past, asthma was treated like a single disease: "Here is your blue inhaler and your brown inhaler." Today, we know asthma is a syndrome—a collection of different diseases that result in the same symptom: wheezing.

We distinguish between:

Phenotype: The observable characteristics (e.g., "Late-onset obese female asthma").

Endotype: The distinct molecular mechanism driving the disease (e.g., "IL-5 driven eosinophilic inflammation").

Precision Medicine: T2-High vs. T2-Low

1. T2-High Asthma (The "Allergic/Eosinophilic" Type) This accounts for about 50-70% of asthma. It is driven by Type 2 inflammation (Th2 cells and ILC2 cells).

Key Cytokines: IL-4, IL-5, and IL-13.

Key Players: Eosinophils, IgE antibodies, and Mast cells.

Response to Steroids: Generally good.

Biologic Targets: This is where we have the most success. Drugs targeting IgE (Omalizumab), IL-5 (Mepolizumab/Benralizumab), and IL-4/13 (Dupilumab) work here.

2. T2-Low Asthma (The "Non-Eosinophilic" Type) This is the harder nut to crack.

Mechanism: Often driven by neutrophils, oxidative stress, or paucigranulocytic (low cell count) processes.

Triggers: Obesity, smoking, pollution, infection.

Response to Steroids: Poor. These patients are often "steroid-resistant."

Therapy: Biologics generally don't work well here yet (as of 2026). Macrolide antibiotics (for anti-inflammatory effect) and bronchial thermoplasty are often considered.

The Biomarker Toolkit

How do you know which type your patient has? You need biomarkers.

Fractional Exhaled Nitric Oxide (FeNO):

Nitric oxide is produced by epithelial cells when they are inflamed by IL-13.

High FeNO (>25-50 ppb): Strongly suggests T2-high/allergic inflammation. It predicts a good response to inhaled steroids.

Blood Eosinophils:

A simple blood count.

High (>150-300 cells/uL): Indicates systemic eosinophilic inflammation. Crucial for qualifying patients for anti-IL-5 therapy.

Total and Specific IgE:

Tells us if the patient is atopic (allergic). Essential for considering anti-IgE therapy.

Occupational Asthma: The Work-Related Wheeze

Occupational Asthma (OA) is the most common form of new-onset asthma in adults. If you miss this diagnosis, you are sending the patient back into a dangerous environment daily.

Two Main Types:

Sensitizer-Induced OA: The immune system develops a specific allergy to a workplace agent.

High-Molecular-Weight (HMW) Agents: Proteins like flour (bakers), animal dander (lab workers), or latex. These usually act via IgE.

Low-Molecular-Weight (LMW) Agents: Chemicals like isocyanates (spray painters), wood dusts, or soldering flux. These act as haptens (they bind to body proteins to become allergenic). They are often IgE-independent and harder to test for.

Irritant-Induced OA: No allergy involved. Caused by a massive exposure to a toxic gas (e.g., chlorine spill). This is often called "Reactive Airways Dysfunction Syndrome" (RADS).

Differentiating "Work-Exacerbated" from "Occupational"
This distinction is legally critical.

Occupational Asthma: The work caused the asthma. (Result: Compensation, job change).

Work-Exacerbated Asthma: The patient already had asthma, but the dusty/cold work environment makes it worse. (Result: Better environmental control, medication adjustment).

The Diagnostic Standard: OASYS You cannot diagnose OA just by history. You need objective data.

Serial Peak Flow Monitoring: The patient measures their lung function every 2 hours while awake, for 4 weeks (2 weeks at work, 2 weeks off work).

OASYS Analysis: A computerized system analyzes this data to see if there is a statistically significant drop in lung function during work periods.

In rare, complex cases, a Specific Inhalation Challenge is performed in a specialized chamber, exposing the patient to the suspected agent under strict medical supervision.

5.3 Biologic Therapies for Respiratory Disease

The revolution in biologics has fundamentally altered the trajectory of severe asthma and Chronic Rhinosinusitis with Nasal Polyps (CRSwNP). As trainees, you must master not just the names of these agents, but the phenotypes they target.

The Landscape: Monoclonal Antibodies

We currently have four major classes of biologics approved for respiratory indications. Understanding their targets is key to matching the right drug to the right patient.

1. Anti-IgE: Omalizumab

Mechanism: Omalizumab binds to free IgE, preventing it from docking onto the FcεRI receptors on mast cells and basophils. It essentially "gums up" the key before it can unlock the allergic cascade.

Status in 2026: It remains the gold standard for severe allergic asthma driven by perennial allergens (dust mites, pets, molds). It is also highly effective for Chronic Spontaneous Urticaria (CSU) and nasal polyps.

2. Anti-IL-5 Pathway: Mepolizumab, Reslizumab, Benralizumab

Mechanism:

Mepolizumab and Reslizumab bind to the IL-5 cytokine itself, neutralizing it.

Benralizumab is unique; it binds to the IL-5 receptor (IL-5Ra) on eosinophils and recruits natural killer cells to destroy them (antibody-dependent cell-mediated cytotoxicity). It basically deletes eosinophils from the blood.

Target Patient: The severe eosinophilic asthmatic. These patients often have late-onset asthma and frequent exacerbations despite high-dose steroids.

3. Anti-IL-4/13: Dupilumab

Mechanism: By blocking the IL-4 receptor alpha subunit, Dupilumab inhibits signaling of both IL-4 and IL-13.

2026 Context: Dupilumab has become a powerhouse for "multi-morbid" Type 2 disease. It treats asthma, severe eczema (atopic dermatitis), and is arguably the most potent agent for shrinking nasal polyps (CRSwNP).

4. Anti-TSLP: Tezepelumab

Mechanism: Tezepelumab targets Thymic Stromal Lymphopoietin (TSLP), an epithelial "alarmin." Think of TSLP as the fire alarm pulled by the airway lining when it encounters smoke, viruses, or allergens. By blocking the alarm, Tezepelumab stops the inflammation before the cascade even starts.

Why it matters: It is the only biologic effective for Type 2-low asthma (non-eosinophilic, non-allergic) because it acts upstream of the Th2 pathway.

Patient Selection and Inclusion Criteria

Selecting a biologic is no longer guesswork; it is algorithm-driven. You must strictly adhere to NICE (UK) or international (GINA/EPOS) guidelines.

Inclusion Checklist (General Principles):

Diagnosis: Confirmed severe asthma (or severe CRSwNP) refractory to optimized standard therapy (high-dose ICS/LABA + LAMA).

Adherence: You must confirm the patient is actually taking their inhalers. Digital inhaler monitoring is now standard practice before starting biologics.

Biomarkers:

Eosinophils: >300 cells/µL favors Anti-IL-5 or Anti-IL-4/13.

FeNO: >25 ppb suggests IL-4/13 driven inflammation (Dupilumab is excellent here).

IgE: Elevated specific IgE favors Omalizumab.

Clinical Pearl: If a patient has severe asthma and massive nasal polyps, Dupilumab or Omalizumab are often preferred over anti-IL-5s because IL-4/13 and IgE are central to polyp growth.

Outcomes: The Shift to "Clinical Remission"

In previous years, we aimed for "control." As of 2026, we aim for remission.

Defining Remission on Biologics:

No Exacerbations: Zero courses of systemic steroids.

No Symptoms: An Asthma Control Questionnaire (ACQ-5) score of < 1.5.

Stable Lung Function: No decline in FEV1.

Biological Silence: Normalization of eosinophils and FeNO.

We also measure outcomes using the SNOT-22 (Sino-Nasal Outcome Test) for polyp patients. A reduction of >8.9 points is considered clinically meaningful, though many patients on biologics see improvements of 30-40 points.

The "Super-Responder" Some patients experience a "Lazarus effect"—their lung function normalizes, and they regain their sense of smell within weeks. These are "super-responders." Conversely, if a patient has not improved after 4-6 months, we must switch agents (e.g., swapping from Anti-IgE to Anti-IL-5).

Safety Profile

Biologics are generally safe, but they are potent immune modulators.

Hypersensitivity: Anaphylaxis is rare (highest with Omalizumab, ~0.1-0.2%) but requires all patients to carry epinephrine pens initially.

Parasitic Infections: IL-5 and IgE are our defense against worms (helminths). Patients traveling to endemic areas need careful counseling. We often screen for Strongyloides before initiation in at-risk groups.

Conjunctivitis: specific to Dupilumab, occurring in ~10-20% of patients (mostly in eczema cohorts, less in asthma).

5.4 Allergen Immunotherapy (AIT) for Respiratory Disease

While biologics block inflammation, Allergen Immunotherapy (AIT) teaches the immune system to ignore the trigger. It remains the only disease-modifying treatment that can alter the natural history of allergic disease.

Mechanisms of Tolerance

How does injecting someone with what they are allergic to actually help them?

The Switch: AIT forces the immune system to shift from a Th2 response (allergic/inflammatory) to a Th1/Treg response (tolerant).

The Block: It induces the production of IgG4 antibodies. These "blocking antibodies" intercept the allergen before it can reach the IgE on the mast cell.

The Peacemakers: It upregulates IL-10 and TGF-beta, anti-inflammatory cytokines that quiet the immune response.

Indications in 2026

Allergic Rhinitis: Moderate-to-severe disease not controlled by antihistamines and nasal steroids.

Allergic Asthma: This is the growth area. Evidence now strongly supports AIT for House Dust Mite (HDM) driven asthma. It reduces exacerbations and steroid load.

Prevention: We now use AIT to prevent the "Atopic March"—stopping a child with hay fever from developing asthma later in life.

Delivery: SCIT vs. SLIT

You will encounter two main modes of delivery in your clinics.

Feature	SCIT (Subcutaneous)	SLIT (Sublingual)
Method	Injections in the clinic.	Tablets/Drops under the tongue at home.
Frequency	Weekly build-up, then monthly maintenance.	Daily.
Key Trials	Historic evidence base.	Grazax (Timothy Grass), Acarizax (Dust Mite).
Safety	Risk of systemic anaphylaxis (requires observation).	Safer; systemic reactions are very rare.
Adherence	High (controlled by doctor).	Variable (patient must remember daily dose).

Pragmatic Considerations: SCIT is labor-intensive. It requires a facility with resuscitation equipment and a waiting room where patients can sit for 60 minutes post-injection. SLIT offloads the labor to the patient but requires discipline.

In 2026, "Cluster Immunotherapy" protocols for SCIT are popular. Instead of coming weekly for months, patients receive multiple injections in a single day to reach maintenance dose faster, though this carries a slightly higher reaction risk.
Logistics of an Immunotherapy Service

Running an AIT clinic is a logistical heavy lift.

Extract Storage: Extracts must be refrigerated and monitored. If the fridge fails, thousands of dollars of stock are lost.

Resuscitation: You cannot administer SCIT without immediate access to IM epinephrine, oxygen, and IV fluids.

Staffing: Specialist nurses are the backbone of these services, monitoring patients for the subtle signs of anaphylaxis (coughing, flushing, itchy palms) during the observation period.

Cutaneous Allergy: Urticaria, Angioedema, and Dermatitis

6.1 Urticaria: Pathogenesis and Management

Introduction: The Evolving Landscape

Urticaria, commonly known as hives, is not merely a skin condition; it is a systemic signal of mast cell dysregulation. By 2026, our understanding has shifted from viewing chronic spontaneous urticaria (CSU) as a singular entity to recognizing it as a spectrum of distinct endotypes. The central player is the mast cell—an immune sentinel that, when triggered, releases a chaotic storm of mediators. While histamine is the most famous of these mediators, it is only the spark; the resulting fire involves a complex interplay of cytokines, leukotrienes, and platelet-activating factors.

Pathophysiology: The Tale of Two Autoimmunities

A critical advancement in the 2026 curriculum is the clear distinction between two pathogenic drivers in CSU. Trainees must move beyond the generic label of "idiopathic" and understand the specific autoimmune mechanisms at play.

1. Type I Autoimmunity (Autoallergic CSU) Think of this as an "allergic reaction to self." In this endotype, the patient produces IgE antibodies not against pollen or peanuts, but against their own endogenous proteins (autoallergens).

Mechanism: Specific IgE antibodies bind to autoantigens such as Interleukin-24 (IL-24) or thyroid peroxidase (TPO). These IgE-antigen complexes then cross-link the FcεRI receptors on mast cells.

Clinical Picture: These patients often present with classic allergic features. They tend to respond rapidly and robustly to Omalizumab (anti-IgE therapy) because the drug mops up the very driver of the disease.

2. Type IIb Autoimmunity (Autoimmune CSU) This is a more aggressive, treatment-resistant form. It accounts for the "hard-to-treat" cases that often frustrate clinicians.

Mechanism: The body produces IgG autoantibodies (not IgE). These IgG antibodies specifically target the IgE receptor itself (FcεRI) or the IgE molecule bound to it. This direct attack activates the complement system and causes massive mast cell degranulation.

Clinical Picture: These patients typically have lower total IgE levels but high basophil activation scores. They often show a poor response to standard antihistamines and even Omalizumab. Historically, they required immunosuppressants like Cyclosporine. However, the 2026 arrival of BTK inhibitors has revolutionized their care.

Chronic Inducible Urticarias (CIndU)

Unlike the spontaneous variety, CIndU has a clear, physical trigger. The mast cells here are "primed" to explode, but they wait for a specific physical signal.

Symptomatic Dermographism: The most common form. Light scratching leads to linear wheals.

Cold Urticaria: Triggered by cold air or water. The risk of anaphylaxis while swimming is a critical safety education point.

Delayed Pressure Urticaria (DPU): Deep, painful swelling occurs 4–6 hours after pressure is applied (e.g., from a tight waistband or carrying a heavy bag). This form is notoriously resistant to antihistamines.

Diagnostic Challenge Testing: Precision diagnosis is mandatory. We no longer rely solely on patient history.

TempTest®: A sophisticated device used to determine the exact temperature threshold for cold or heat urticaria.

FricTest: A standardized friction test for dermographism. Knowing the threshold allows patients to manage their daily lives—for example, knowing they are safe at 15°C but at risk at 10°C.

Management: The 2026 Stepwise Algorithm

The management of urticaria has become a model of precision medicine. The "trial and error" days are over. We follow a strict escalation protocol based on the EAACI/GA²LEN/EDF/WAO guidelines.

Step 1: Second-Generation H1-Antihistamines We start with non-sedating antihistamines (e.g., bilastine, fexofenadine). First-generation agents (like diphenhydramine) are obsolete in chronic management due to their cognitive side effects. They are the "rotary phones" of allergy medicine—functional but outdated.

Step 2: Up-Dosing (Four-Fold) If standard dosing fails after 2–4 weeks, we do not switch drugs immediately. Instead, we escalate the dose up to four times the standard daily limit. This high-dose strategy saturates the H1 receptors, providing relief for about 50-60% of patients.

Step 3: Biologics (Omalizumab) For those still suffering (refractory cases), Omalizumab remains a cornerstone. It acts as a "chemical sponge," soaking up free IgE. In 2026, biosimilar versions have made this more accessible, though it remains a high-cost intervention.

Step 4: The Game Changer – BTK Inhibitors (Remibrutinib) This is the most significant update in the 2026 edition.

The Drug: Remibrutinib (Rhapsido®).

The Mechanism: It inhibits Bruton's Tyrosine Kinase (BTK). BTK is an enzyme inside the mast cell that acts as a central signal relay. By blocking BTK, Remibrutinib essentially "cuts the power cord" to the mast cell.

Why it Matters: Unlike Omalizumab, which targets IgE (Type I), Remibrutinib blocks the intracellular signaling pathway. This means it works for both Type I (autoallergic) and Type IIb (autoimmune) urticaria. It is an oral tablet, offering a massive quality-of-life improvement over injectable biologics. Clinical data from the REMIX-1 and REMIX-2 trials demonstrated rapid symptom control, often within the first week.

Step 5: Immunosuppression (Cyclosporine) With the advent of BTK inhibitors, Cyclosporine is now relegated to a last-resort option due to its renal toxicity and hypertension risks.

Monitoring: Trainees must use the UAS7 (Urticaria Activity Score over 7 days). This patient-reported outcome measures the number of wheals and intensity of itch. A score of 0 is the target: complete freedom from disease.

6.2 Angioedema: Hereditary and Acquired

Introduction: The Silent Threat

Angioedema is swelling of the deep dermis and subcutaneous tissues. While it often co-occurs with urticaria, isolated angioedema is a red flag. The clinician's primary duty is to distinguish between two mechanisms:

Histaminergic: Associated with hives and itch. Responds to antihistamines and adrenaline.

Bradykinin-Mediated: No hives. No itch. Does not respond to adrenaline or antihistamines. This is the killer. Misdiagnosing a bradykinin attack as an allergic reaction can be fatal if the airway is involved.

Hereditary Angioedema (HAE): A Genetic Storm

HAE is a rare, autosomal dominant disorder caused by a deficiency or dysfunction of C1-Inhibitor (C1-INH). Without this "brake," the plasma kallikrein-kinin system runs wild, overproducing bradykinin. Bradykinin increases vascular permeability, causing fluid to leak into tissues.

Classification:

Type I: Low levels of C1-INH protein (85% of cases).

Type II: Normal levels, but the protein is dysfunctional (15% of cases).

HAE with Normal C1-INH (Type III): The C1-INH levels and function are normal. The fault lies elsewhere. Recent genetic sequencing has identified mutations in Factor XII, Plasminogen, Angiopoietin-1, and Kininogen-1.

Therapeutic Management: The 2026 Paradigm Shift

The goal in 2026 is "Zero Attacks." We have moved from managing crises to preventing them entirely.

1. Acute "On-Demand" Treatment Every patient must have an emergency plan. If a laryngeal attack occurs, standard allergy meds are useless.

Icatibant (Firazyr): A bradykinin B2 receptor antagonist. It blocks the receptor that bradykinin tries to bind to. Administered subcutaneously.

C1-INH Concentrates (Berinert, Ruconest): Intravenous replacement of the missing protein.

2. Long-Term Prophylaxis (LTP) This area has seen explosive innovation. The old standard, Danazol (an attenuated androgen), is now largely historical due to side effects like virilization and liver toxicity.

Oral Kallikrein Inhibitors: Berotralstat (Orladeyo). A once-daily pill that inhibits plasma kallikrein. It has liberated patients from the burden of injections, offering a "normal life" oral regimen.

Monoclonal Antibodies: Lanadelumab (Takhzyro). This antibody binds to and inhibits plasma kallikrein. Administered every 2 to 4 weeks, it provides highly effective, steady-state protection.

New in 2026 - Garadacimab (Andembry): The first monoclonal antibody targeting activated Factor XII (Factor XIIa). By hitting the cascade higher upstream than kallikrein inhibitors, it offers potent monthly prophylaxis via autoinjector.

New in 2026 - RNA-Targeted Therapy: Donidalorsen (Dawnzera). This is a precision medicine marvel. It is an antisense oligonucleotide (ASO) that targets the RNA responsible for producing Prekallikrein (PKK). By reducing the production of the precursor protein, it prevents the cascade from ever starting. Dosed monthly or every two months, it has shown near-total suppression of attacks in Phase 3 trials (OASIS-HAE).

3. The Frontier: Gene Editing We are currently witnessing the dawn of a cure.

CRISPR/Cas9 (NTLA-2002): This in vivo gene-editing therapy is designed to be a "one-and-done" treatment. It uses lipid nanoparticles to deliver CRISPR machinery to the liver. The machinery edits the KLKB1 gene (which produces prekallikrein) directly inside the patient's cells, permanently knocking it out. Early data shows a 95-97% reduction in angioedema attacks after a single infusion. This represents the transition from "chronic management" to "functional cure."

6.3 Atopic Dermatitis and Systemic Therapy

The Pathophysiology: The "Leaky Wall" and the "Fire"

To treat Atopic Dermatitis (AD), you must understand the "dual-hit" hypothesis. Imagine the skin as a brick wall. The "bricks" are corneocytes (skin cells), and the "mortar" is the lipid bilayer that seals them together.

In many AD patients, this wall is genetically defective. A key mutation occurs in the Filaggrin gene. Filaggrin is a protein that bundles keratin filaments to create a tough structural barrier. When Filaggrin is absent or mutated, the skin cells collapse like a deflationary balloon. Water escapes (Transepidermal Water Loss), and allergens get in. This is the "Leaky Wall."

Once the barrier is breached, the immune system reacts. This is the "Fire." The breach activates the innate immune system, releasing "alarmins" (TSLP, IL-25, IL-33). These alarms wake up Type 2 Innate Lymphoid Cells (ILC2) and Th2 lymphocytes.

These cells flood the tissue with specific cytokines:

IL-4 and IL-13: These destroy the barrier further and increase inflammation.

IL-31: This is the "itch cytokine." It directly stimulates nerve endings, causing the patient to scratch. Scratching breaks the barrier more, letting in more allergens. This is the itch-scratch cycle.

In 2026, we now also recognize the role of Th22 and Th17 pathways in specific subtypes of eczema, particularly in Asian populations and pediatric patients. This heterogeneity explains why one drug doesn't work for everyone.

Clinical Skill: The Allergy Detective

A major pitfall for trainees is the "Food Allergy Trap." Parents of infants with eczema are often desperate. They see the skin flaring and assume it must be something the baby ate.

You must differentiate sensitization from allergy.

In infants with moderate-to-severe eczema, the gut is often healthy, but the skin is leaky. Food proteins (peanut, egg, milk) present in house dust land on the broken skin. The immune system sees these proteins through the skin and builds IgE antibodies against them. This is sensitization. It means the blood test is positive, but the child might actually tolerate the food if they eat it.

However, if you tell the parents to remove that food from the diet based solely on a blood test, you may cause a disaster. By removing the food from the gut (where tolerance is learned) while the skin exposure continues, you can convert a harmless sensitization into a life-threatening anaphylactic allergy.

The Golden Rule for 2026: Never order a "food panel" indiscriminately for eczema. Only test for foods if there is a history of immediate reaction (hives, vomiting) within minutes of ingestion. For infants with severe eczema, early introduction of peanuts and eggs is the standard of care to prevent allergy, not avoidance.

The Therapeutic Ladder (2026 Update)

We treat eczema in steps. We do not jump to biologics immediately.

Step 1: Barrier Repair (The Foundation) Every patient gets this. We use liberal emollients to replace the missing "mortar." In 2026, we also use "prescription device" creams that mimic physiological lipids (ceramides, cholesterol, fatty acids in a 3:1:1 ratio).

Step 2: Anti-Inflammatory Topicals (The Fire Extinguishers)

Topical Steroids: Still the gold standard for flares. We use them intermittently to put out the fire.

Topical Calcineurin Inhibitors (Tacrolimus): Safe for the face and eyelids where steroids cause thinning.

The "New" Non-Steroidals:

Roflumilast (PDE4 Inhibitor): A once-daily cream that blocks inflammation without steroid side effects.

Tapinarof (AhR Agonist): Another steroid-free cream that helps restore the barrier while stopping inflammation.

Ruxolitinib Cream (Topical JAK): Approved for short-term use. It is incredibly potent, often working as fast as a strong steroid, but systemic absorption is low.

Step 3: Systemic Therapy (The Heavy Artillery) When topicals fail, we move to systemics. In the past, we used broad immunosuppressants like Methotrexate or Cyclosporine. These were "blunt instruments" that suppressed the whole immune system. Today, we use "smart bombs"—Biologics and Small Molecules.
Biologics: The Monoclonal Antibodies

These are large proteins, injected subcutaneously. They target outside the cell.

Dupilumab (Dupixent): The pioneer. It blocks the receptor for IL-4 and IL-13. It is safe, effective, and requires no blood monitoring. It is the baseline against which all others are measured.

Tralokinumab (Adbry) & Lebrikizumab (Ebglyss): These are pure IL-13 blockers. By sparing IL-4, they offer a slightly different mechanism. Lebrikizumab has a high binding affinity, allowing for monthly dosing after the induction phase.

Nemolizumab (Nemluvio): The newest game-changer for 2025/2026. It targets the receptor for IL-31 (the itch cytokine). It is unique because it stops the itch almost immediately, often before the rash fully clears. For patients where sleep disturbance and scratching are the dominant symptoms, this is the drug of choice.

Side Effects of Biologics: They are generally safe. The most common side effect is Conjunctivitis (red, itchy eyes). This is manageable with eye drops and rarely requires stopping the drug.

JAK Inhibitors: The Small Molecules

These are oral pills (Upadacitinib, Abrocitinib). Unlike biologics, which block the cytokine outside the cell, JAK inhibitors enter the cell and block the signal inside the nucleus.

They are the "sprinters." They work faster than biologics, often clearing skin in days. They are incredibly powerful. However, they are less specific. They block the JAK-STAT pathway, which is used by many body systems.

The Safety Monitoring Protocol: Because they are systemic, we must monitor for safety.

Venous Thromboembolism (VTE): There is a slight risk of blood clots. We avoid these in patients with a history of clots or heavy smokers.

Herpes Zoster (Shingles): JAK inhibitors can wake up the chickenpox virus. In 2026, we vaccinate all patients against Shingles (Shingrix) before starting these drugs.

Infections: We monitor for tuberculosis and serious infections.

Labs: We check Complete Blood Count (CBC), Liver enzymes, and Lipids (cholesterol) every 3-4 months.

6.4 Contact Dermatitis and Patch Testing

The Mechanism: Type IV Hypersensitivity

Contact Dermatitis is different from hives. It is not an immediate histamine release. It is a Type IV Delayed Hypersensitivity reaction.

Here is the timeline:

Induction: The chemical (hapten) penetrates the skin. It binds to a skin protein. Dendritic cells grab it and take it to the lymph node. They teach T-cells to hate this chemical. This takes weeks.

Elicitation: The patient touches the chemical again. Nothing happens immediately. But 24 to 48 hours later, those trained T-cells march into the skin and release inflammatory cytokines. The skin swells, blisters, and itches.

This delay is why patients are confused. They say, "I put on the cream on Monday, but the rash didn't start until Wednesday. It can't be the cream!" You must explain that this delay is the hallmark of the disease.

The Diagnostic Tool: Patch Testing

We cannot diagnose this with a blood test. We must reproduce the disease in a controlled setting. This is the Patch Test.

The Methodology:

Day 0 (Monday): We apply small chambers containing allergens to the patient's healthy back skin. We tape them down. The patient cannot shower or sweat.

Day 2 (Wednesday): We remove the tape. We look at the skin. Often, it looks normal because of the pressure of the tape. We wait.

Day 4 (Friday): This is the critical reading. The skin has recovered from the tape pressure, and the delayed immune reaction is peaking.

Reading the Results:

Negative (-): Normal skin.

Irritant (IR): The skin looks burned or glazed, but not allergic. This happens with soaps or acids. It does not spread.

Allergic (+ to +++): Redness, infiltration (bumpy feel), and vesicles (blisters). The reaction often spreads beyond the square of the chamber.

The Allergens: What are we testing?

In 2026, we use the European Baseline Series (Updated) as our starting point. This contains the roughly 30 most common allergens in our environment.

1. The Metals:

Nickel: The most common allergen worldwide. Found in cheap jewelry, belt buckles, and even coins.

Cobalt & Chromium: Often found in leather tanning (shoes) and cement.

2. The Preservatives:

Methylisothiazolinone (MI): This was the "allergen of the decade" a few years ago. It is used in water-based paints, wet wipes, and shampoos. Regulations have lowered the allowed concentrations, but we still see highly sensitized patients.

Formaldehyde Releasers: Chemicals that slowly release formaldehyde to kill bacteria in cosmetics.

3. The Fragrances:

We test Fragrance Mix I and Fragrance Mix II.

In 2026, we also pay close attention to Limonene and Linalool hydroperoxides. These are natural citrus and lavender oils. When they are fresh, they are safe. But when they oxidize (sit on a shelf exposed to air), they turn into potent allergens. "Natural" does not mean safe.

4. The Paediatric Baseline (2026 Standard): We now have a standardized series for children (pEBS). It includes 18 specific allergens. We test kids for things like Tixocortol-21-pivalate (a marker for steroid allergy) and Propolis (bee glue used in "natural" balms).

Occupational Dermatitis and Hand Eczema

Occupational skin disease is a major economic burden. A hairdresser who is allergic to hair dye cannot work. A mechanic allergic to grease is disabled.

We use Occupational Series based on the job:

Hairdressing Series: Tests for PPD (hair dye) and Ammonium Persulfate (bleach).

Bakery Series: Tests for flour enzymes and spices.

Epoxy Series: For construction workers and wind turbine engineers.

The Hand Eczema Revolution: For years, chronic hand eczema (CHE) was a graveyard of treatment failures.

Food Allergy: Diagnosis, Management, and Nutrition

7.1 IgE-Mediated Food Allergy Across the Lifespan

The Pediatric vs. Adult Paradigm Shift

Historically, we viewed food allergy as a childhood disease that one might "outgrow." In 2026, we recognize it as a lifelong dynamic condition. The "Classic 8" allergens (milk, egg, peanut, tree nut, fish, shellfish, wheat, soy) still dominate pediatrics, but the presentation is changing.

Pediatric Presentation: In infants, the immune system is learning to distinguish "self" from "non-self." When this process fails, we see immediate reactions—hives (urticaria), vomiting, and wheezing—often to ubiquitous proteins like casein (milk) or ovalbumin (egg).

2026 Update: We now see that early introduction (the "prevention window" between 4-6 months) has successfully reduced peanut allergy prevalence, yet we are seeing a rise in "persistent" milk and egg allergies that do not resolve by age five.

Adult-Onset Allergy: This is the new frontier. A patient who has eaten shrimp their entire life suddenly develops anaphylaxis at age 45. Why?

Mechanism: Loss of oral tolerance. This is often driven by environmental changes or gut microbiome dysbiosis.

Key Allergens: In adults, the primary culprits are shellfish (tropomyosin), finfish (parvalbumin), and increasingly, seeds (sesame, flax).

Clinical Vignette: Consider "Sarah," a 32-year-old architect. She eats a bagel with hummus and develops laryngeal edema (throat swelling). It isn't the chickpea; it's the sesame (tahini). In 2026, sesame is firmly established as a major adult allergen, often requiring clearer labeling than in previous decades.

The Tale of Two Fruits: PFAS vs. LTPs

One of the most critical skills for an ACI (Allergy and Clinical Immunology) physician is distinguishing between Pollen Food Allergy Syndrome (PFAS) and Lipid Transfer Protein (LTP) allergy. They both involve reactions to fruits and vegetables, but one is a nuisance, and the other is a killer.

1. Pollen Food Allergy Syndrome (PFAS) / Oral Allergy Syndrome

This is a class example of "molecular mimicry." The immune system is sensitized to a pollen (usually Birch tree pollen, Bet v 1). The proteins in certain raw fruits (apples, cherries, peaches) look structurally similar to the pollen.

The "Cooked Apple" Test: This is the diagnostic key. The protein involved (homologues of Bet v 1) is heat-labile. It falls apart when cooked.

Scenario: A patient says, "My mouth itches when I eat a raw Granny Smith apple, but I can eat apple pie just fine." This is PFAS. The risk of systemic anaphylaxis is extremely low because the stomach acid destroys the protein before it enters the blood.

2. Lipid Transfer Protein (LTP) Allergy: The "Mediterranean" Phenotype

LTPs are the plant's defense proteins—they are designed to be tough. They withstand heat, cold, and low pH.

The Danger: Unlike PFAS, if a patient is allergic to the LTP in a peach (Pru p 3), they cannot eat peach jam, peach juice, or roasted peaches. The protein survives the stomach, enters the bloodstream, and can cause systemic shock.

The "Cofactor" Effect: In 2026, we pay heavy attention to "cofactors." A patient might tolerate a peach on a lazy Sunday. But if they eat a peach and then go for a jog (Exercise) or take ibuprofen (NSAID), their threshold drops, and they anaphylax. This is "Cofactor-Augmented Anaphylaxis."

Alpha-gal Syndrome: The "Midnight Anaphylaxis"

Alpha-gal (Galactose-alpha-1,3-galactose) is unique because it is an allergy to a carbohydrate, not a protein.

The Vector: The Lone Star Tick (Amblyomma americanum). In Ireland and the UK, we are also watching the Ixodes tick populations closely as vectors shift with climate change.

The Mechanism: A tick bites the human, injecting alpha-gal sugar into the blood. The body creates IgE against this sugar. Later, the human eats mammalian meat (beef, pork, lamb), which is rich in alpha-gal.

The Delay: Unlike a peanut reaction (minutes), Alpha-gal reactions take 3-6 hours. This delay occurs because the sugar is bound to fats (glycolipids), which take longer to digest and enter the circulation.

2026 Clinical Insight: We now screen for Alpha-gal in cases of "idiopathic anaphylaxis." If a patient wakes up at 2:00 AM in shock, ask about their dinner (steak?) and their hobbies (hiking/tick exposure?).

Diagnostic Precision: Component-Resolved Diagnostics (CRD)

In 2026, we rarely rely on "whole extract" testing alone. We use CRD to look at the specific molecular components.

Peanut Example:

Ara h 2: Storage protein. High risk of anaphylaxis. Strict avoidance needed.

Ara h 8: Pollen-related protein (birch cross-reactivity). Low risk. The patient can likely tolerate peanut butter but might get an itchy mouth.

Impact: This distinction prevents unnecessary dietary restrictions, improving the patient's quality of life.

7.2 Non-IgE Mediated Food Allergy: The Gastrointestinal Spectrums

We now shift gears to the "slow" allergies. These do not involve histamine; they involve T-cells and eosinophils attacking the gut lining. Standard skin prick tests (which measure IgE) are negative here, making diagnosis a challenge of clinical acumen.

Food Protein-Induced Enterocolitis Syndrome (FPIES)

FPIES is often called "sepsis-like allergy" because the infant looks incredibly sick—pale, lethargic, and hypotensive—but has no hives.

The Acute Presentation: An infant eats oat cereal. Two hours later, they begin projectile vomiting (15-20 times). They become floppy and blue. In the ER, they are often misdiagnosed with a viral stomach bug or sepsis.

The Trigger: Historically, we thought of milk and soy. In 2026, we recognize rice and oats as the predominant solid-food triggers in FPIES.

Adult FPIES: We are seeing more documented cases in adults, particularly triggered by mollusks (clams, oysters) and crustaceans. The symptoms are intense abdominal cramping and vomiting, often mistaken for food poisoning.

Management: Strict avoidance. There is no EpiPen for FPIES (epinephrine works on IgE/histamine pathways). The treatment for an acute attack is IV fluids to combat hypovolemic shock and IV ondansetron (Zofran) to stop the vomiting.

Eosinophilic Esophagitis (EoE): The Dysphagia Crisis

EoE is a chronic allergic inflammation of the esophagus. The esophagus, which should be a smooth muscular tube, becomes stiff, ringed, and furrowed due to eosinophilic infiltration.

Symptoms by Age:

Infants: Refusal to feed, spit-up.

Children: Abdominal pain, vomiting.

Adults: Dysphagia (trouble swallowing) and food impaction (steak getting stuck).

Diagnostic Criteria:

You must have biopsies.

Threshold: >15 eosinophils per high-power field (hpf) on microscopy, persisting despite PPI therapy (though the PPI requirement has softened in the 2025 guidelines).

The 2026 Management Algorithm (The "3-D" Approach):

Diet: The "Six-Food Elimination Diet" (Milk, Egg, Wheat, Soy, Nut, Seafood) is effective but hard to maintain. The "Step-Up" approach (starting by just removing milk and wheat) is now preferred to increase compliance.

Drugs (Topical Steroids): Swallowed fluticasone or budesonide slurry. It coats the esophagus to reduce inflammation locally.

Dupilumab (Biologics): This is the game-changer. As of 2026, Dupilumab (targeting IL-4 and IL-13 pathways) is standard therapy for severe, refractory EoE in adults and children (aged 1+). It targets the underlying type 2 inflammation directly, often allowing patients to liberalize their diet.

The Role of the ACI Physician in 2026

The allergist is no longer just a "skin tester." You are a coordinator of care.

In EoE: You work with gastroenterologists to time endoscopies with dietary reintroductions.

In FPIES: You work with dietitians to ensure the infant gets adequate nutrition despite excluding major food groups.

In IgE: You risk-stratify patients for new therapies like oral immunotherapy (OIT) or biologic prophylaxis (Omalizumab), which allows patients to tolerate accidental exposures.

7.3 Diagnostic Food Challenges: The Gold Standard

The Oral Food Challenge (OFC) remains the definitive test for diagnosing food allergy. Despite advances in component-resolved diagnostics (CRD) and basophil activation tests (BAT), the OFC is the only tool that replicates the real-world physiological response to ingestion. It is, in essence, a controlled risk procedure. Your role is to balance diagnostic clarity with patient safety.

Protocol Architectures: Open, Single-Blind, and DBPCFC

We classify challenges based on "blinding"—who knows what the patient is eating.

1. Open Food Challenge: This is the workhorse of clinical practice. Both the clinician and the patient (or parent) know what food is being ingested.

Utility: It is most efficient for confirming tolerance (a "ruled-out" allergy) or for confirming allergy in young children where psychological factors are minimal.

Limitation: In older children and adults, anxiety can manifest as subjective symptoms (nausea, lump in throat), creating false positives.

2. Single-Blind Food Challenge: Here, the patient is unaware of whether they are eating the allergen or a placebo, but the clinician knows. This reduces patient bias but leaves room for observer bias—where you, the clinician, might subconsciously over-interpret a mild cough because you know the patient just ate peanut.

3. Double-Blind Placebo-Controlled Food Challenge (DBPCFC): This is the gold standard for research and complex clinical cases. Neither the patient nor the clinician knows the content of the challenge meal.

The Procedure: The challenge is split into two days. One day involves the active allergen; the other involves a placebo matrix (masking vehicle).

The Matrix: Creating a convincing placebo is an art form. For a peanut challenge, we often use a vehicle like apple sauce, chocolate pudding, or a lentil-based patty to mask the texture and smell of roasted peanut flour. If a patient reacts on the "active" day but tolerates the "placebo" day, the diagnosis is confirmed. If they react on both, the symptoms are likely psychological or coincidental.

Risk Stratification: Setting the Scene

Before a single crumb is ingested, you must "risk-stratify" your patient. This determines where the challenge happens.

Low-Risk (Outpatient Clinic): Consider a 12-month-old with a low sIgE to egg who has never reacted but has severe eczema. This child is unlikely to have a life-threatening airway collapse. A standard clinic room with basic resuscitation equipment (adrenaline, oxygen) is sufficient.

High-Risk (Day-Case Unit): Consider a 15-year-old with asthma and a history of trace-exposure anaphylaxis to cashew. This patient requires a high-dependency setting. You need IV access established before the challenge starts, continuous pulse oximetry, and a team ready for full resuscitation.

Critical Example: Never challenge a patient with uncontrolled asthma. If their FEV1 (forced expiratory volume) is below 80% predicted, the challenge is contraindicated. Asthma is the single biggest risk factor for fatal anaphylaxis during a challenge.

The Procedure: Dosing and Stopping Rules

A standard OFC is a marathon, not a sprint. We use a semi-logarithmic incremental dosing schedule.

Starting Dose: We begin with a "no-effect" dose, often 1 mg to 3 mg of protein.

Progression: Doses are doubled every 15 - 20 minutes (e.g., 3mg → 10mg → 30mg → 100mg → 300mg → 1g → 3g).

Goal: The target is usually a cumulative dose of 4–6 grams of protein, which represents an age-appropriate serving size (e.g., a full glass of milk or two tablespoons of peanut butter).

Interpretation: The Pass, The Fail, and The Grey Area

The Pass (Negative): The patient eats the full serving with no symptoms. They remain under observation for at least 2 hours post-challenge to ensure no delayed reaction occurs. Next Step: The patient must incorporate the food into their diet immediately to maintain tolerance.

The Fail (Positive): Objective symptoms appear. These are undeniable signs: urticaria (hives), angioedema (swelling), vomiting, wheezing, or hypotension.

Action: Stop the challenge immediately. Treat with antihistamines for cutaneous symptoms or intramuscular adrenaline for respiratory/cardiovascular compromise.

The Grey Area: This is where your skill is tested. A patient complains of an "itchy tongue" or "tummy ache" at dose 4. Are they reacting? Or are they anxious?

Strategy: Do not stop. Do not treat. Wait. Pause the protocol for 30 minutes. If symptoms resolve, repeat the same dose. If symptoms escalate to objective signs (e.g., one hive becomes three), the challenge is positive. If they disappear, proceed.

7.4 Prevention and Immunotherapy: The Paradigm Shift

As of 2026, the landscape of food allergy management has shifted entirely from "passive avoidance" to "active immune modulation." We no longer just tell patients what not to eat; we teach them how to retrain their immune systems.

Primary Prevention: The 2026 ASCIA/BSACI Guidelines

The most significant public health victory in our field has been the standardization of early introduction. The 2026 guidelines (building on the LEAP and EAT studies of the previous decade) are unequivocal:

The Window of Opportunity: Tolerance induction is most effective between 4 and 6 months of age. Delaying introduction beyond 12 months significantly increases the risk of developing an allergy.

Protocol for High-Risk Infants: For infants with severe eczema or existing egg allergy, we do not wait.

Peanut: Introduce smooth peanut butter (thinned with breast milk or warm water) at 4–6 months. Never use whole nuts (choking hazard).

Egg: Introduce well-cooked egg (hard-boiled or baked) initially. Raw or lightly cooked egg (scrambled) is more allergenic and should be introduced only after baked egg is tolerated.

The "Once-is-Not-Enough" Rule: A common parental mistake is feeding the allergen once, seeing no reaction, and then not feeding it again for weeks. The guidelines emphasize regularity. To maintain the tolerant state, the infant must consume the allergen at least 2–3 times per week consistently throughout the first years of life.

Oral Immunotherapy (OIT): Treatment, Not Cure

For those who have already established an allergy, OIT is the primary therapeutic option. As of 2026, we utilize both licensed products (like Palforzia for peanut) and standardized off-label hospital protocols for milk, egg, and walnut.

Mechanism of Action: You must distinguish between two clinical states:

Desensitization: This is the temporary raising of the reaction threshold. While on daily therapy, the patient can eat 300mg of peanut (roughly one kernel) without reacting. This protects against accidental exposure.

However, if they miss a dose for 3-4 days, the protection collapses, and they are at risk of anaphylaxis again.

Sustained Unresponsiveness (SU) / Remission: This is the "Holy Grail." It implies that the patient can stop daily dosing for weeks or months and still consume the food safely. Currently, SU is harder to achieve and typically requires years of therapy.

Protocols (e.g., Palforzia): OIT follows a three-phase architecture:

Initial Escalation (ID): A single day in a high-dependency unit. We start at micro-doses (e.g., 0.5 mg) and rapidly updose to 6 mg under strict supervision.

Build-Up Phase: Every two weeks, the patient returns to the clinic to step up the dose (e.g., 6mg → 12mg → 20mg...). In between visits, they take the current safe dose daily at home.

Maintenance: Once the target (usually 300mg to 3000mg) is reached, the patient continues this daily indefinitely.

Managing the Burden and Safety (The "Dark Side" of OIT): OIT is not a free lunch. It exchanges the potential risk of accidental reaction for the certainty of minor reactions and daily burden.

Adverse Events: Most patients will experience oral itching or mild abdominal pain during the build-up. Systemic reactions (anaphylaxis) can occur, often triggered by "cofactors."

The Cofactor Rule: A dose that is safe at breakfast might cause anaphylaxis if taken right before a gym class (exercise), during a viral infection, or during menstruation. Patients must be educated to "downtitrate" or skip doses during these high-risk windows.

Eosinophilic Esophagitis (EoE): This is the most significant long-term complication. Approximately 5–10% of OIT patients develop EoE—a chronic, allergic inflammation of the esophagus causing dysphagia (difficulty swallowing) and food impaction.

Surveillance: If a patient on OIT reports "food sticking" in the chest or chronic heartburn, you must stop therapy and refer for endoscopy. Unlike IgE-mediated reactions, EoE is slow-onset and does not respond to adrenaline.

Drug Allergy and Hypersensitivity

8.1 Beta-Lactam Allergy and De-labelling

The Problem: The "90% Fake News" Label

If you walk into any hospital ward today, you will see "Penicillin Allergy" written on red wristbands everywhere. It is the most common drug allergy label in the world. However, the data tells a shocking story: fewer than 10% of these patients are truly allergic.

Why does this happen? Usually, a child has a viral rash while taking amoxicillin. The parents assume it is an allergy, the doctor writes it down to be safe, and that label sticks for life.

In 2026, we view this label not just as a nuisance, but as a patient safety risk. Patients with an incorrect penicillin allergy label are:

Given broad-spectrum antibiotics (like Vancomycin or Ciprofloxacin) which are more toxic.

More likely to develop superbugs like C. difficile or MRSA.

Subject to longer hospital stays.

Therefore, de-labelling—the process of removing this incorrect label—is now a core competency (Specialty CiP 1) for all trainees.

Risk Stratification: The "Traffic Light" System

We cannot test everyone in a specialist clinic; there are simply too many patients. The solution is Risk Stratification.

This means sorting patients into groups based on their history to decide who needs a specialist and who can be tested safely on the ward.

1. Low Risk (Green Light)

Who are they? Patients who had a rash (not hives) more than 10 years ago, or patients who only experienced side effects like nausea or headache.

The 2026 Approach: These patients do not need skin testing. The skin test is painful, expensive, and can actually give false positives.

Action: We proceed straight to a Direct Oral Challenge (DOC). This means giving the patient a single dose of amoxicillin (usually 250mg or 500mg) and watching them for one hour.

Service Model: In modern hospitals, this is often a "nurse-led" or "pharmacist-led" service. A specialist does not need to be in the room, provided a doctor is nearby.

2. Moderate Risk (Amber Light)

Who are they? Patients with a history of urticaria (hives) or an itchy rash that happened recently (less than 10 years ago).

The Risk: There is a small but real chance they still have IgE antibodies.

Action: These patients require Skin Testing (skin prick and intradermal tests) first. If the skin test is negative, we then proceed to the oral challenge.

3. High Risk (Red Light)

Who are they? Anyone with a history of:

Anaphylaxis: Throat closing, wheezing, collapse.

SCAR (Severe Cutaneous Adverse Reactions): This includes Stevens-Johnson Syndrome (SJS) or DRESS syndrome. These are blistering skin diseases that can be fatal.

Action: Do not challenge. These patients require strict avoidance and specialist evaluation. We never perform oral challenges on patients with a history of blistering skin reactions.

Setting Up a De-labelling Service

As a trainee, you may be asked to design a de-labeling pathway. The "2026 Standard" is the Point-of-Care Model.

In the past, we referred everyone to the allergy clinic. Now, we bring the test to the patient. For example, a pharmacist reviewing a patient's chart on the Orthopedic ward notices a "Penicillin Allergy" label. They take a quick history. If it sounds "Low Risk," they get approval to give the test dose right there on the ward (with consent).

Evidence Base: Recent large-scale studies (2024-2025) have shown that Direct Oral Challenge in low-risk patients is incredibly safe. The rate of severe reaction is near zero. Even if a rash occurs, it is usually mild and easily treated with antihistamines.

8.2 Perioperative and General Anaesthetic Hypersensitivity

The Nightmare Scenario

Imagine this: A patient is on the operating table. The anaesthetist induces sleep. Suddenly, the heart rate shoots up, the blood pressure crashes to unrecordable levels, and the lungs become impossible to ventilate.

This is Perioperative Anaphylaxis. It is a "high-stakes" emergency because the patient is unconscious and cannot tell you "my throat feels tight." It is purely a physiological storm.

In the UK and Europe, the incidence is roughly 1 in 10,000 surgeries. While that sounds rare, it is often life-threatening. The latest National Audit Project (NAP7) reports confirm that Neuromuscular Blocking Agents (NMBAs) and Antibiotics remain the top two killers.

The Suspects

When a reaction happens, the patient has usually received 5 or 6 drugs at once. Our job as allergists is to be the detective and find the culprit.

1. Neuromuscular Blocking Agents (NMBAs)

Drugs like Rocuronium and Suxamethonium are muscle relaxants used to help intubate the patient.

The Problem: They are the most common cause of anaphylaxis in anaesthesia.

Cross-Reactivity: The structural part of the drug that causes the allergy is the "Quaternary Ammonium Ion." Unfortunately, this ion is present in almost all muscle relaxants. This means if a patient is allergic to Rocuronium, they might also be allergic to Vecuronium or Atracurium.

Testing: We use skin prick testing and intradermal testing. However, skin tests for NMBAs are tricky; they can irritate the skin and cause "false positives." We have to be very careful with our interpretation.

2. Antibiotics

Co-amoxiclav (Augmentin) and Teicoplanin are frequently given right before the knife cuts to prevent infection.

Teicoplanin is becoming a more frequent trigger. It is often used in patients labeled with penicillin allergy—another reason why de-labelling (Section 8.1) is so important!

3. Chlorhexidine: The "Hidden" Enemy

This is the silent threat. Chlorhexidine is an antiseptic used to clean the skin, but it is also hidden on:

Central venous catheters (coated tips).

Lubricant gels (for urinary catheters).

The 2026 Update: We now routinely screen for Chlorhexidine in unexplained anaphylaxis because the anaesthetist might not even realize they administered it (e.g., the surgeon used a coated catheter).

4. Patent Blue Dyes

Used in breast cancer surgery to find lymph nodes. These can cause severe anaphylaxis, often delayed by 30-60 minutes.

The Investigation Pathway

Timing is everything. You cannot test the patient immediately after the reaction because their immune system is "depleted."

Immediate Phase (In the Operating Room):

Take a Mast Cell Tryptase blood test immediately. Tryptase is an enzyme released by exploding mast cells.

Take a second sample 1-2 hours later.

Take a baseline sample 24 hours later.

The Rule: A sharp rise in tryptase confirms anaphylaxis. If the tryptase stays flat, it might have been a non-allergic event (like sepsis or overdose).

The Clinic Visit (4-6 Weeks Later):

We wait at least 4 weeks for the mast cells to "recharge."

Skin Testing: We perform skin prick tests for all drugs given. If negative, we perform Intradermal Tests (injecting a tiny amount under the skin).

The Challenge of Specific IgE: Blood tests (Specific IgE) are available for Penicillin and Suxamethonium, but for many drugs (like Propofol or newer opiates), reliable blood tests simply do not exist.

New Frontiers: BAT and MAT (The 2026 Perspective)

What happens if the skin tests are negative, but the story sounds like a severe allergy? In 2026, we are increasingly using cellular tests:

BAT (Basophil Activation Test): We take the patient's live blood cells and expose them to the drug in a test tube. If the cells "light up" (express markers like CD63), the patient is allergic.

MAT (Mast Cell Activation Test): Similar to BAT but uses mast cells. These tests are becoming vital for complex cases, especially for NMBAs where skin tests can be inconclusive.

The Output: The Safe Anaesthetic Plan

The final and most important step is the letter you write to the anaesthetist. It is not enough to say "Allergic to Rocuronium." You must provide a Safe Plan.

Example of a Safe Plan:

"This patient had confirmed anaphylaxis to Rocuronium. Cross-reactivity testing shows she is safe to use Cisatracurium. She is also safe to use Propofol and Fentanyl. Please avoid all Chlorhexidine products as a precaution until further testing confirms safety."

You must also ensure the patient wears a MedicAlert bracelet. In the digital age of 2026, we also upload this "Safe Plan" directly to the patient's national electronic health record so that if they are in a car accident, the emergency team knows exactly what drugs to avoid.

8.3 Severe Cutaneous Adverse Reactions (SCARs)

Overview Welcome to the advanced module on SCARs. In 2026, we view these not just as "rashes," but as systemic, T-cell mediated immunological storms. They are medical emergencies. The mortality rate remains significant, but our ability to predict and treat them has improved drastically over the last five years.

The three major phenotypes you must recognize are Stevens-Johnson Syndrome (SJS), Toxic Epidermal Necrolysis (TEN), and Drug Reaction with Eosinophilia and Systemic Symptoms (DRESS/DiHS).

Pathophysiology: The T-Cell Storm

These reactions are delayed hypersensitivity (Type IV). They are not caused by antibodies (IgE) but by T-cells that have gone rogue.

The Mechanism: A specific drug binds to a Human Leukocyte Antigen (HLA) receptor on your cells. The immune system mistakes this drug-protein complex for a foreign invader.

Cytotoxic Attack: CD8+ cytotoxic T-cells release death signals—granulysin and perforin. These proteins punch holes in the skin cells (keratinocytes), leading to massive cell death.

Genetic Keys: We now know that genetics load the gun.

HLA-B*58:01: Strongly linked to Allopurinol (gout medication).

HLA-B*57:01: Linked to Abacavir (HIV medication).

HLA-B*51:02: Update: This is a critical association for Osimertinib (a lung cancer drug) widely recognized in Asian populations.

Clinical Phenotypes & Diagnosis

1. SJS and TEN Think of these as burns from the inside out. The difference is the extent of skin detachment.

SJS: Less than 10% of body surface area.

SJS/TEN Overlap: 10–30%.

TEN: Greater than 30%.

Diagnostic Tools:

ALDEN Score: We use this algorithm to mathematically determine which drug is the culprit.

SCORTEN vs. CRISTEN: While SCORTEN predicts mortality, the newer CRISTEN score is increasingly used in 2026 to stratify risk based on renal and respiratory function earlier in the disease course.

Biopsy: Mandatory. You will see "full-thickness necrosis" of the epidermis.

2. DRESS (DiHS) This is the "great mimicker." It affects the skin, but it kills through organ failure.

The Triad: Fever, Eosinophilia (high white blood cells), and Organ Involvement (Liver/Kidney/Heart).

Viral Reactivation: A unique feature of DRESS is that it often wakes up dormant viruses like HHV-6 (Human

Herpesvirus 6). This leads to a "stuttering" course where symptoms flare up even after the drug is stopped.

Management Strategy (2026 Protocols)

Phase 1: The Acute Phase (Survival)

Stop the Drug: This is the single most effective action. Every hour of continued exposure increases mortality.

Supportive Care: Treat like a burn victim. Fluid replacement, temperature control, and high-protein nutrition.

Adjuvant Therapies:

Cyclosporine: A powerful calcineurin inhibitor. It stops the T-cells from releasing death signals. It is now a standard first-line choice for SJS/TEN.

Biologics (The New Standard): In 2026, we frequently use Etanercept (TNF-alpha inhibitor) for TEN to block inflammation. For DRESS with severe eosinophilia, we use IL-5 inhibitors like Mepolizumab or Benralizumab.

JAK Inhibitors: Drugs like Tofacitinib are showing promise in refractory DRESS cases.

Phase 2: The Convalescent Phase (Prevention)

Contraindication: The patient must never take the drug again.

In-Vitro Testing: Re-challenging the patient (giving the drug again) is dangerous. Instead, we use the Lymphocyte Transformation Test (LTT) or ELISPOT.

How it works: We take the patient's blood and expose their white blood cells to the drug in a test tube. If the cells multiply (transform), the drug is confirmed as the culprit. This is safe and effective.

8.4 Chemotherapy Desensitization

Overview Cancer patients often develop allergies to their life-saving chemotherapy (Platinums, Taxanes) or Monoclonal Antibodies (mAbs). In the past, we had to stop treatment. Today, we use Rapid Drug Desensitization (RDD).

Principles of RDD

RDD is not a cure for allergy. It is a "temporary truce."

Mechanism: We trick the mast cells. By introducing the drug in microscopic amounts and slowly increasing the dose, we lock the mast cells in an unresponsive state.

Critical Rule: Tolerance lasts only as long as the drug is in the blood. If the patient misses a dose, the allergy returns. The process must be repeated for every single cycle.

Protocols: The "Bag" System

We mix the drug into different concentrations (bags) to prevent accidental overdose.

3-Bag Protocol (Standard):

- Bag A: 1% of the total dose.
- Bag B: 10% of the total dose.
- Bag C: 100% of the total dose.

Procedure: We infuse Bag A very slowly, then faster. Then switch to Bag B, and finally Bag C. This takes 4–6 hours.

4-Bag Protocol (High Risk): Used for patients who have had severe anaphylaxis. We add a "Bag Very Dilute" (0.1% concentration) to start even slower.

One-Bag Protocol: Emerging in some centers to save pharmacy time, but it carries a higher risk of error if the pump is not programmed perfectly.

Advanced Management: Phenotypes & Biomarkers

Not all reactions are simple allergies. We now distinguish between two main types to guide treatment.

1. Type I Hypersensitivity (Classic Allergy)

Symptoms: Hives, flushing, throat closing.

Biomarker: Elevated Tryptase levels.

Treatment: RDD is highly effective.

2. Cytokine Release Syndrome (CRS)

Symptoms: Fever, chills, rigorous shaking, muscle pain. Common with monoclonal antibodies (like Rituximab) and oxaliplatin.

Biomarker: Elevated Interleukin-6 (IL-6).

Treatment: RDD may not work alone. We often add Tocilizumab (an IL-6 blocker) or steroids to the premedication protocol.

Clinical Competency: Managing Breakthroughs

A "breakthrough" is when the patient reacts during the desensitization.

Step 1: Stop the infusion immediately.

Step 2: Treat the reaction (Antihistamines for hives, Epinephrine for hypotension).

Step 3: Once stable, restart the infusion at the previous safe step.

Step 4: Do not abandon the procedure unless the reaction is life-threatening (Grade 4). Most patients can finish the dose with adjustments.

Insect Venom and Occupational Allergy

9.1 Hymenoptera Venom Allergy

Natural History and Epidemiology

Hymenoptera venom allergy is a classic IgE-mediated disease, yet its expression is remarkably variable. In the general population, sensitization (presence of specific IgE) is common—up to 25% of adults may have positive skin tests—yet only a fraction of these individuals will experience systemic anaphylaxis upon a sting.

The culprit insects generally fall into two families: Apidae (honeybees, bumblebees) and Vespidae (wasps, yellow jackets, hornets). The behavior of the insect often dictates the clinical picture. Honeybees (Apis mellifera) are usually docile and sting only when provoked, leaving the barbed stinger and venom sac in the skin. Vespids (Vespula, Polistes), however, are aggressive scavengers with smooth stingers, capable of inflicting multiple stings in a single attack.

Clinical Presentations: The Great Divide

Trainees must learn to rigorously differentiate between Large Local Reactions (LLR) and Systemic Anaphylaxis. This distinction determines the therapeutic trajectory.

Large Local Reactions (LLR): These are characterized by swelling exceeding 10 cm in diameter that persists for more than 24 hours. While alarming to the patient—sometimes encompassing an entire limb—an LLR is generally not a risk factor for future anaphylaxis. The risk of progression to a systemic reaction in LLR patients is low (around 5-10%), and VIT is rarely indicated.

Systemic Anaphylaxis: This involves symptoms remote from the sting site. We utilize the Ring and Messmer grading system to classify severity, ranging from Grade I (generalized urticaria) to Grade IV (cardiovascular collapse/arrest).

Clinical Pearl: In children, strictly cutaneous systemic reactions (Grade I) have a benign natural history, with a very low risk (<10%) of progression to severe anaphylaxis on subsequent stings. Conversely, adults with even mild systemic reactions carry a much higher risk of progression.
Diagnostic Precision: Navigating the "Double-Positive" Trap

One of the most frequent challenges in the clinic is the patient who tests positive for both honeybee and wasp venom. Is this true double sensitization (bad luck), or is it cross-reactivity?

In 2026, we rely heavily on Component-Resolved Diagnostics (CRD) to solve this puzzle.

Whole venom extracts contain Cross-Reactive Carbohydrate Determinants (CCDs). These are sugar moieties found on venom proteins (like hyaluronidase) that are shared across species—and even shared with plant pollens. Many patients develop IgE antibodies against these sugars (anti-CCD IgE), which are clinically irrelevant but cause positive test results for both bee and wasp venom in vitro.

To cut through this noise, we test for specific recombinant allergens (molecular components) that are species-specific and usually free of CCDs:

Honeybee (Apis): Look for sensitization to Api m 1 (Phospholipase A2). This is the marker of genuine honeybee sensitization.

Wasp (Vespula): Look for sensitization to Ves v 1 (Phospholipase A1) and Ves v 5 (Antigen 5).

Polistes (Paper Wasp): Look for Pol d 5.

If a patient is "double positive" on whole venom but only positive to Ves v 5 (and negative to Api m 1), they are allergic to wasps, and the bee result was a false positive due to CCDs. Treating this patient with bee venom immunotherapy would be unnecessary and unethical.

The Mastocytosis Connection

Perhaps the most critical safety lesson in this module is the link between venom allergy and Clonal Mast Cell Disorders (MCD). Hymenoptera venom is a potent mast cell secretagogue. In patients with an underlying surplus of mast cells (mastocytosis), a sting can trigger catastrophic, hypotensive anaphylaxis that is resistant to epinephrine.

Screening Protocol:

Baseline Tryptase: Every patient with a history of systemic sting reaction must have a baseline serum tryptase measured (ideally >24 hours after the reaction).

Thresholds: A baseline level >11.4 ng/mL is the traditional flag. However, current 2026 guidelines emphasize that any elevated tryptase in the context of hypotensive syncope (Grade IV reaction) warrants investigation.

Bone Marrow Biopsy: Trainees should use tools like the REMA score to decide when to refer for a bone marrow biopsy. Patients with absence of urticaria/angioedema (the "silent shock" phenotype) and elevated tryptase are at highest risk for systemic mastocytosis.

9.2 Venom Immunotherapy (VIT)

Venom Immunotherapy is the only disease-modifying treatment available for insect allergy. It is highly effective, offering protection rates of 95-98% for wasp allergy and roughly 80-90% for bee allergy. The lower efficacy in bee allergy is likely due to the higher allergen content in bee venom and the sensitizing nature of the sting delivery.

Mechanism of Action

VIT works by shifting the immune response from a Th2-driven allergic profile (high IL-4, IL-13) to a regulatory Th1/T-reg profile. The hallmark of success is the induction of Venom-Specific IgG4. These "blocking antibodies" intercept the venom proteins before they can cross-link IgE on the surface of mast cells, effectively neutralizing the trigger.

Indications for Therapy

Who should receive VIT?

Adults: Indicated for Systemic Reactions (Grade II-IV) involving respiratory or cardiovascular symptoms. For mild Grade I reactions (skin only), VIT is optional and depends on Quality of Life (QoL)—e.g., a patient who is terrified to go outdoors.

Children: Indicated for moderate-to-severe systemic reactions (respiratory/cardiovascular). VIT is generally NOT indicated for children with cutaneous-only reactions, as their spontaneous remission rate is high.

Induction Protocols: The Need for Speed

The goal of the induction phase is to reach the maintenance dose (usually 100 µg of venom, equivalent to ~2 stings) safely.

Conventional Protocol: Injections are given weekly for 3-6 months. This is slow and leaves the patient unprotected for a long duration.

Rush and Ultra-Rush Protocols: In 2026, these are increasingly the standard of care in specialized centers.

Rush: Reaches maintenance in 3-5 days.

Ultra-Rush: Reaches maintenance in a single day (e.g., 3.5 hours).

Ultra-rush protocols typically involve hospital admission for safety monitoring but are highly cost-effective. They rapidly restore Quality of Life, allowing the patient to leave the hospital fully protected. Pre-medication with antihistamines is standard to reduce side effects.

Duration of Therapy: When to Stop?

The "Standard of Care" has long been a 3 to 5-year course of monthly injections. Discontinuing VIT after 5 years results in long-term tolerance for most patients. However, "most" is not "all."

Indefinite (Lifelong) Therapy: Certain high-risk groups should never stop VIT:

Mastocytosis / Elevated Tryptase: These patients have a high relapse rate and the risk of fatal reactions remains elevated.

Severe Initial Reaction: Patients who experienced near-fatal cardiac arrest (Grade IV) before treatment.

Honeybee Allergy with High Exposure: Beekeepers often require ongoing therapy due to the intense, repeated exposure and lower efficacy of bee VIT.

9.3 Occupational Lung and Skin Disease

The Medicolegal Interface

Occupational disease is unique because it sits squarely at the intersection of clinical medicine and statutory law. In 2026, the physician's role has evolved from merely treating symptoms to acting as a pivotal detective in a legal framework. When a worker develops asthma or dermatitis due to their job, it is not just a health issue; it is potentially a compensable injury and a failure of workplace safety protocols.

Diagnosing an occupational condition requires a mindset shift. You are no longer asking just "What does the patient have?" but rather "What did the patient breathe or touch, and when?" The implications of a positive diagnosis are profound: the patient may lose their livelihood, the employer may face legal action under regulations like RIDDOR (Reporting of Injuries, Diseases and Dangerous Occurrences Regulations), and the workplace may require expensive engineering overhauls.

Clinical Example: Consider "Elias," a 45-year-old spray painter. He presents with worsening wheeze. If you diagnose "adult-onset asthma" and prescribe an inhaler, you treat the symptom. If you diagnose "isocyanate-induced occupational asthma," you trigger a cascade of events: Elias is removed from exposure, his employer must report the case to the health and safety executive, and his colleagues are screened. The latter approach saves lives; the former merely palliates.

Occupational Asthma: The Two Pathways

Occupational asthma (OA) remains the most frequently reported occupational respiratory disease in industrialized nations. As of the 2026 guidelines, we categorize causative agents into two distinct groups based on their molecular size, as this dictates the immune mechanism and the clinical presentation.

1. High Molecular Weight (HMW) Agents (>5-10 kDa) These are typically biological proteins. The immune system identifies them as foreign invaders and mounts a classic Type I Hypersensitivity response. This involves the production of specific IgE antibodies.

Mechanism: IgE-mediated.

Latency: Sensitization takes time. A worker may handle flour for five years without issue, then suddenly develop symptoms.

Clinical Phenotype: Recent 2025 cohort studies indicate that HMW asthma is strongly associated with "warning signs" like work-related rhinitis (sneezing/runny nose) and conjunctivitis (itchy eyes) before the chest symptoms start.

Common Culprits:

Flour: The scourge of bakers. Fungal alpha-amylase (an additive) is often the specific allergen.

Laboratory Animals: Rat and mouse urinary proteins are potent sensitizers.

Seafood: Aerosolized proteins from crab or prawn processing.

2. Low Molecular Weight (LMW) Agents (<1 kDa) These are chemicals, too small to be recognized by the immune system on their own. They act as "haptens," binding to the body's own proteins (like albumin) to form a new, immunogenic complex.

Mechanism: Often uncertain. While some act via IgE, many LMW agents drive asthma through non-IgE pathways, possibly involving T-lymphocytes.

Clinical Phenotype: Unlike HMW agents, LMW agents often lack the "warning" nasal symptoms. They are associated with isolated chest tightness and, worryingly, a higher risk of severe exacerbations (asthma attacks) compared to HMW agents.

Common Culprits:

Isocyanates: Found in spray paints, foams, and glues. Despite "green" initiatives, they remain the leading cause of OA in the automotive sector.

Persulfates: Bleaching agents used by hairdressers.

Wood Dusts: Western Red Cedar (plicatic acid).

The Diagnostic Algorithm (2026 Protocol)

The diagnosis of OA cannot rely on history alone. Workers often conflate "feeling bad at work" with true immunological reactions. The gold standard remains objective confirmation using the OASYS plotting system.

Step 1: Serial Peak Flow Measurements The trainee must instruct the patient to perform Peak Expiratory Flow (PEF) readings. The 2026 standard is strict:

Frequency: At least 4 times per day (waking, mid-day, evening, bed).

Duration: Minimum of 3 weeks, encompassing periods at work and periods away from work (holidays or weekends).

Technology: Modern digital spirometers now upload data directly to the cloud, allowing the OASYS software to analyze the diurnal variation instantly.

Step 2: OASYS Analysis The software looks for the "occupational effect"—a pattern where lung function progressively deteriorates during the work week and recovers during rest days. A score of >2.5 on the OASYS index is highly specific for occupational asthma.

Step 3: Immunological Testing

Skin Prick Testing / Specific IgE: useful only for HMW agents. You can test for flour or latex allergy. You generally cannot blood test for an isocyanate allergy reliably.

Specific Inhalation Challenge: The patient is exposed to the suspect agent in a controlled, hospital-based booth. This is the "reference standard" but is expensive, risky, and reserved for complex medico-legal disputes.

Occupational Dermatitis

Skin disease accounts for a massive burden of occupational morbidity. We distinguish two main types:

Irritant Contact Dermatitis (ICD):

Cause: Direct physical or chemical damage to the skin barrier. No immune memory is involved. Anyone exposed to enough strong acid or wet-work will get this.

Appearance: Dry, cracked, fissured hands. Often confined strictly to the area of contact.

Example: A nurse washing hands 40 times a day, stripping away the lipid layer.

Allergic Contact Dermatitis (ACD):

Cause: A Type IV (delayed) T-cell mediated hypersensitivity.

Appearance: Vesicular (blistered), weeping, red rash. Can spread beyond the point of contact.

Diagnostic Test: Patch Testing (reading at 48 and 96 hours).

Example: A construction worker sensitized to chromates in wet cement.

The Hierarchy of Controls Managing occupational skin and lung disease requires a rigid hierarchy. Physicians must not jump straight to PPE.

Elimination: Stop using the toxic agent. (e.g., stopping the use of powdered latex gloves).

Substitution: Replace a toxic chemical with a safer one (e.g., using water-based paints instead of isocyanate-based ones).

Engineering Controls: Install local exhaust ventilation (LEV) to suck fumes away from the worker's breathing zone.

Administrative Controls: Rotate workers to reduce exposure time.

PPE (Personal Protective Equipment): The last resort. Respirators and gloves rely on perfect user compliance, which is rarely achieved.

9.4 Latex Allergy

The 2026 Landscape

In the 1990s, latex allergy was an epidemic. By 2026, the prevalence has stabilized, but it has not vanished. While most Western healthcare systems have moved to "latex-free" environments, the risk has shifted to other sectors (cleaning, food handling, and hair/beauty) and remains a critical issue for patients with multiple surgeries.

We also see a phenomenon of "re-emergence" in supply chains. During global disruptions, lower-quality latex products with high protein content occasionally flood the market, re-sensitizing workers who had been safe for years.

Pathophysiology and Risk Groups

Natural Rubber Latex (NRL) comes from the Hevea brasiliensis tree. The sap contains proteins (Hev b 1 through Hev b 13) that serve as defense mechanisms for the plant. Unfortunately, these proteins are potent allergens for humans.

High-Risk Groups:

Healthcare Workers (HCWs): Despite improvements, sensitization rates in some regions hover around 5-10%.

Spina Bifida Patients: This is the most tragic group. Due to repeated surgeries (shunt revisions, bladder repairs) starting from infancy, up to 70% of spina bifida patients are sensitized to latex. For them, a latex reaction can be anaphylactic and fatal.

Rubber Industry Workers: Those manufacturing tires or condoms.

Latex-Fruit Syndrome

This is a fascinating example of molecular mimicry. The proteins in latex (specifically Hev b 6, the prohevein) are structurally almost identical to defense proteins found in certain plants. If the body's antibodies learn to attack latex, they may mistakenly attack these foods.

The "Classic" Offenders:

Banana

Avocado

Kiwi

Chestnut

The "New" Offenders (2026 Updates): Recent literature has expanded this list. We now recognize Zucchini (Courgette) and Turnip as emerging triggers for Latex-Fruit syndrome.

Clinical Insight: A patient who reports an itchy mouth (Oral Allergy Syndrome) when eating a banana should be flagged immediately. Do not use latex gloves for their catheterization. The "banana" allergy is the red flag for a potential anaphylactic reaction to latex during surgery.

Management Strategies

There is no cure for latex allergy; immunotherapy remains experimental and risky. Management is purely defensive.

1. The Latex-Safe Environment For a sensitized patient (e.g., spina bifida), the operating theater must be "latex-safe."

Protocol: No powdered gloves anywhere in the room (powder binds latex protein and makes it airborne).

Equipment: Syringe plungers, vial stoppers, and IV tubing must be verified non-latex.

Timing: These patients should be the first case of the day. This ensures that any aeroallergens (latex particles floating in the air) from the previous day have settled or been vented out by the HVAC system.

2. Personal Avoidance For the occupationally allergic worker, "low-protein" gloves are often not enough. Complete avoidance is required. This often necessitates a career change or a rigorous enforcement of glove-free policies for the entire department, as the worker can react to the particles shed by a colleague's gloves standing five feet away.

Primary Immunodeficiency: Antibody and Cellular Defects

10.1 Predominantly Antibody Deficiencies

The Context: The "Bread and Butter" of Adult Immunology

When you enter an adult immunology clinic, antibody deficiencies will be your most frequent companion. Unlike the dramatic, early-onset immune failures of infancy, these conditions often lurk in the background for years. A patient might tell you they are "just prone to colds," or they have a "bad chest." It is your job to recognize the pattern in the noise.

The hallmark of these disorders is a failure of the B-cell arm of the immune system. B-cells are the factories. Their product is immunoglobulin (antibody). When the factories shut down, or when they produce defective goods, the body loses its primary defense against extracellular bacteria.

Common Variable Immunodeficiency (CVID): The Great Mimic

Defining the Undefined CVID is not a single disease. In 2026, we view it as a "clinical bucket"—a collection of different genetic defects that all result in a similar crash of the immune system. It is a diagnosis of exclusion. You cannot diagnose CVID if there is another cause (like lymphoma, medication use, or a known single-gene defect).

To label a patient with CVID, we look for three things:

Hypogammaglobulinemia: A significant reduction in IgG, usually combined with low IgA and/or IgM.

Functional Impairment: It is not enough to have low numbers. The antibodies must fail to work. We prove this by vaccinating the patient (e.g., with Pneumovax) and seeing no response.

Clinical Consequence: Recurrent infections or immune dysregulation.

The Two Roads of CVID Clinically, CVID patients tend to diverge down one of two paths. Understanding this dichotomy is critical for prognosis.

The "Infectious" Phenotype: About roughly half of CVID patients stay in this lane. Their life is dominated by susceptibility to encapsulated bacteria. They suffer from recurrent otitis media, sinusitis, and pneumonia. If untreated, this leads to bronchiectasis—a permanent scarring and widening of the airways that traps mucus and breeds further infection.

Example: Consider "John," a 35-year-old accountant. He has had pneumonia three times in the last two years. Between episodes, he has a chronic cough. His CT scan shows thickened bronchial walls in the lower lobes. He has no other symptoms. This is the classic infectious phenotype. His treatment is straightforward: replace the missing immunoglobulins.

The "Inflammatory" or "Complex" Phenotype: This is the more dangerous road. In these patients, the immune system is not just weak; it is confused. It attacks the self. In 2026, we recognize that CVID is as much a disease of immune dysregulation as it is of deficiency.

Autoimmunity: These patients frequently destroy their own blood cells. You might see autoimmune hemolytic anemia (AIHA) or immune thrombocytopenia (ITP). Paradoxically, a patient who cannot make antibodies to fight pneumonia might make auto-antibodies that destroy their own platelets.

Granulomas: The immune system tries to wall off perceived threats, forming clumps of cells called granulomas in the lungs, skin, or liver. This can mimic Sarcoidosis.

Enteropathy: A CVID gut can look identical to Celiac disease, with blunted villi and chronic diarrhea, but it does not respond to a gluten-free diet.

GLILD (Granulomatous-Lymphocytic Interstitial Lung Disease): This is a specific, aggressive lung complication where lymphocytes flood the lung tissue.

Example: Consider "Sarah," age 28. She has low IgG, but she rarely gets pneumonia. Instead, she presents with a massive spleen (splenomegaly), low platelets, and swollen lymph nodes. A biopsy of her nodes shows benign hyperplasia, not cancer. She represents the inflammatory phenotype. Giving her immunoglobulin replacement will stop infections, but it will not fix her swollen spleen or autoimmunity. She needs immune suppression (like corticosteroids or targeted biologics) alongside her immune replacement.

Specific Antibody Deficiency (SAD): The Invisible Defect

SAD is a diagnosis that requires high suspicion. These patients have normal levels of Immunoglobulins (IgG, IgA, IgM are all normal). However, the quality of the antibody is poor.

Specifically, they cannot build a defense against polysaccharide antigens. Bacteria like Streptococcus pneumoniae are coated in a sugar (polysaccharide) capsule. This capsule is slippery; the immune system needs to tag it with specific antibodies to grab it. Patients with SAD fail to make antibodies against these sugars.

Diagnosis and Management We diagnose this by "challenging" the immune system. We measure antibody levels against pneumococcus, give the Pneumovax vaccine, and measure again 4-6 weeks later. A SAD patient will show a "flat" response—no rise in titers.

Clinical Management: Many patients with mild SAD can be managed with prophylactic antibiotics (e.g., Azithromycin three times a week) to keep the bacterial load down. If infections persist and lungs begin to scar, we escalate to Immunoglobulin replacement therapy (IgRT), just like in CVID.

10.2 Severe Combined Immunodeficiency (SCID) and T-cell Defects

The Pediatric Emergency

If CVID is a slow-burning fire, SCID is an explosion. It is the most severe form of Primary Immunodeficiency. The definition is in the name: "Combined" refers to the loss of both T-cell and B-cell function.

T-cells are the conductors of the immune orchestra. Without T-cells, B-cells cannot function (even if they are present). Therefore, a T-cell defect is effectively a total immune collapse.

The Presentation: Failure to Thrive In the era before newborn screening, these infants presented at 3 to 6 months of age. As maternal antibodies (transferred via placenta) faded, the infant was left defenseless.

The Pattern: A baby who is not gaining weight ("failure to thrive") and suffers from opportunistic infections.

The Pathogens: These are not just normal colds. These are infections that healthy babies fight off easily. Pneumocystis jirovecii pneumonia (PCP), severe fungal thrush that spreads down the esophagus, and disseminated viral infections (like CMV or Rotavirus) are typical.

Newborn Screening: The Game Changer

By 2026, widespread adoption of the TREC assay in newborn screening has revolutionized outcomes.

How it works: When a T-cell is made in the thymus, it rearranges its DNA to build a receptor. This cutting and pasting of DNA produces a waste product: a small circle of DNA called a TREC (T-cell Receptor Excision Circle).

The Logic: A healthy baby has millions of naive T-cells, so they have high TREC counts. A baby with SCID is not making T-cells, so their TREC count is near zero. This allows us to catch these babies before they get sick, which doubles their survival rate.

Immunological Phenotypes and Genetics

We classify SCID based on which lymphocytes are missing. This helps us guess the genetic mutation.

T- B+ NK- SCID (The Common Form):

The Defect: T-cells are absent. B-cells are present (but useless). Natural Killer (NK) cells are absent.

The Gene: Usually the Common Gamma Chain (IL2RG) mutation. This is X-linked, meaning it affects boys. The gamma chain is a shared part of the receptors for several cytokines (IL-2, IL-4, IL-7, etc.) that tell cells to grow. Without it, the cells starve.

T- B- NK+ SCID (The Metabolic Form):

The Defect: Both T-cells and B-cells are missing. NK cells are present.

The Gene: Often Adenosine Deaminase (ADA) deficiency or RAG1/RAG2 deficiency. In ADA deficiency, toxic metabolites build up inside the lymphocytes and poison them.

T- B- NK- SCID (The Total Absence):

The Gene: Reticular Dysgenesis (very rare).

Management Strategy: Bridge to Cure

SCID is fatal without treatment. Management is a race against time.

Phase 1: Immediate Protection (The "Bridge") Once SCID is suspected (e.g., a positive TREC test), the infant is a medical emergency.

Isolation: The infant must be kept in a positive-pressure, HEPA-filtered room. No live vaccines (like Rotavirus or BCG) can be given—these would be lethal.

Prophylaxis: We start medications immediately to prevent PCP pneumonia (Trimethoprim-Sulfamethoxazole) and antifungals.

Ig Replacement: Since the baby cannot make antibodies, we infuse IVIG (intravenous immunoglobulin) to provide passive immunity.

Phase 2: Definitive Cure There are two main paths to a cure in 2026.

Hematopoietic Stem Cell Transplantation (HSCT): This remains the standard. We replace the baby's defective bone marrow with healthy marrow from a donor.

Best Scenario: An HLA-identical sibling donor. Survival is >90%.

Alternative: A haploidentical parent (half-match) or matched unrelated donor. Conditioning chemotherapy is often required to "make space" for the new marrow, but this carries toxicity risks.

Gene Therapy (GT): In 2026, Gene Therapy has moved from experimental to a first-line option for specific types like ADA-SCID and X-linked SCID.

The Process: We harvest the baby's own stem cells. In a lab, we use a viral vector (usually a lentivirus) to insert a correct copy of the missing gene into the cells. We then infuse the corrected cells back into the baby.

The Advantage: No risk of Graft-versus-Host Disease (GVHD) because the cells are the baby's own. The immune system is restored without attacking the body.

Module 10.3: Combined Immunodeficiencies (CID)

Overview: The "Middle Ground" of Immunity

We often think of immunodeficiency as a black-and-white issue: either you have an immune system, or you don't (like in Severe Combined Immunodeficiency, or SCID). But Combined Immunodeficiencies (CIDs) exist in the gray area. They are the "leaky" phenotypes. In these conditions, T and B cells are present but functionally impaired. The engine runs, but it sputters.

Unlike SCID, where infants present with life-threatening infections in the first months of life, CID patients often have a more insidious course. They might survive infancy but struggle with a lifetime of "weird" complications—not just infections, but also autoimmunity and cancer. This module explores the classic syndromes you must recognize in 2026.

1. Hyper-IgE Syndromes (Job's Syndrome)

Historically called "Job's Syndrome" (after the biblical figure plagued by boils), this category has split into two distinct genetic entities as of the mid-2020s. You must learn to distinguish them, as the management is radically different.

A. Autosomal Dominant Hyper-IgE (STAT3 Deficiency)

Think of this as a disorder of tissue structure and immune signaling. The STAT3 mutation breaks the pathway for IL-17, a cytokine critical for defending mucosal barriers (skin and lungs) and remodeling bone.

The Clinical Picture: These patients often have a very specific "look" (coarse facies). The hallmark is the "Cold Abscess." They get massive staphylococcal boils on the skin that feel squishy but lack the heat and redness of normal inflammation because their immune system doesn't mount a "hot" response.

The Lung Trap: Recurrent pneumonias lead to pneumatoceles (air-filled cysts). . If a fungal infection (like Aspergillus) gets into these cysts, it is catastrophic.

Skeletal Features: Because STAT3 is involved in bone health, these patients have retention of primary teeth (baby teeth don't fall out), scoliosis, and fragile bones.

B. Autosomal Recessive Hyper-IgE (DOCK8 Deficiency)

This is the "viral" cousin. While they also have high IgE and eczema, their problem is a failure of cytoskeletal reorganization in immune cells. T cells cannot "squeeze" through tissues to get to the virus.

The Viral Storm: Unlike STAT3 patients, DOCK8 patients are ravaged by cutaneous viruses. You will see severe, spreading Molluscum contagiosum, massive HPV warts, and severe Herpes Simplex/Zoster.

Malignancy Risk: This is critical for your 2026 practice: DOCK8 deficiency carries a high risk of skin cancers and lymphomas, often driven by these unchecked viruses. Early Hematopoietic Stem Cell Transplant (HSCT) is curative and recommended here, whereas it is controversial in STAT3.

2. Wiskott-Aldrich Syndrome (WAS)

WAS is an X-linked disorder affecting the actin cytoskeleton of blood cells. The platelets are small, and the immune cells can't form the "synapse" needed to talk to each other.

The Classic Triad (EXIT):

Eczema (often severe and bleeding).

Immunodeficiency (recurrent ear/sinus infections).

Thrombocytopenia (low platelets).

Important: The platelets in WAS are microthrombocytes (tiny platelets). This distinguishes it from ITP (Immune Thrombocytopenic Purpura), where platelets are large.

2026 Update: The Gene Therapy Era For decades, HSCT was the only cure. However, late 2025 saw the landmark FDA and EMA approval of etuvetidigene autotemcel (Waskyra). This autologous gene therapy uses a lentiviral vector to insert a correct copy of the WAS gene into the patient's own stem cells. It effectively "reprograms" their immune system without the risk of Graft-versus-Host Disease (GvHD). For trainees in 2026, WAS is no longer just a transplant disease; it is a gene therapy disease.
3. Ataxia-Telangiectasia (A-T)

A-T is a DNA repair defect (mutation in the ATM gene). The body cannot repair double-strand DNA breaks. This affects cells that divide rapidly (immune cells) or are biologically complex (neurons).

The Clinical Trap: The "Ataxia" (wobbly gait) usually starts before the "Telangiectasia" (dilated eye vessels). A toddler presenting with wobbly walking is often misdiagnosed with cerebral palsy. The telangiectasias might not appear until age 3-5.

Immunology: Variable. Some have low IgA/IgG, others are normal.

Radiosensitivity: Never expose these patients to unnecessary X-rays or CT scans. Their DNA cannot repair the damage, leading to massive cancer risks (leukemia/lymphoma).

4. Non-Infectious Manifestations: The "Dysregulation"

In CID, the immune system is not just weak; it is confused. About 30-50% of your workload with these patients will be managing immune dysregulation, not infections.

Autoimmunity: The remaining T cells may attack the host. Autoimmune Cytopenias (attacking own blood cells) are common in partial RAG deficiency.

Granulomas: In CIDs, the immune system can't clear a pathogen, so it "walls it off" instead, forming granulomas in the skin, liver, or lungs.

Malignancy: A surveillance program is mandatory. The lack of "tumor surveillance" by T and NK cells predisposes these patients to lymphomas.

Module 10.4: Diagnostic Approach to Recurrent Infections
The "Infection-Prone" Patient

As an immunologist, 90% of the referrals you receive for "recurrent infections" will turn out to be normal children or adults with secondary issues. Your job is to find the needle in the haystack without bankrupting the healthcare system.

The "Rule of Too": When taking a history, look for infections that are:

Too Frequent: (e.g., >2 pneumonias in a year).

Too Severe: (e.g., needing IV antibiotics, ICU admission).

Too Prolonged: (e.g., requiring 3 courses of antibiotics to clear).

Too Unusual: (e.g., Burkholderia or Aspergillus in a non-hospitalized patient).

Differentiation: PID vs. Secondary Causes

Before ordering genetic panels, rule out the "Big Three" masqueraders:

Anatomical Defects: A child with recurrent meningitis might have a skull fracture or sinus defect, not an immune problem. Recurrent pneumonia in the same lobe suggests a foreign body or malformation.

Atopy (Allergy): Allergic rhinitis causes mucosal swelling, trapping bacteria. These kids have "recurrent sinusitis" because they are allergic, not immunodeficient. Treating the allergy stops the infection.

Secondary Immunodeficiency: In 2026, medication-induced immunosuppression (biologics, steroids) is the #1 cause of secondary ID. Always review the drug chart.

The Diagnostic Hierarchy (2026 Framework)

We move in tiers. Do not jump to Tier 3 unless the phenotype is severe (e.g., failure to thrive + severe pneumonia).

Tier 1: The Screen (The "GP" Level)

Full Blood Count (FBC): Look for neutropenia (low neutrophils) or lymphopenia (low lymphocytes). Pearl:

SCID babies have low lymphocytes. Never ignore lymphopenia in an infant!

Immunoglobulins (IgG, IgA, IgM, IgE): Quantitative levels.

Vaccine Responses: This is a functional test. We measure antibodies to Tetanus or Pneumococcus. If the patient was vaccinated but has zero antibodies, their B cells are "present but lazy" (Specific Antibody Deficiency).

Tier 2: The Phenotype (The "Specialist" Level)

Lymphocyte Subsets (Flow Cytometry): We count the T cells (CD3, CD4, CD8), B cells (CD19), and NK cells (CD16/56). This tells us who is missing.

Complement Studies (CH50/AH50): For patients with recurrent meningitis or sepsis.

Tier 3: The Deep Dive (The "Tertiary" Level)

Functional Assays: Tests like DHR (for Chronic Granulomatous Disease) or Lymphocyte Proliferation studies (do the T cells blast when stimulated?).

Genetics: In 2026, Rapid Whole Genome Sequencing (rWGS) is becoming the standard for acutely ill infants. For outpatients, targeted panels (Next-Generation Sequencing) remain cost-effective.

Immune Dysregulation and Innate Immunity Disorders

Chronic Granulomatous Disease (CGD)

The "Broken Blast" Mechanism Imagine a soldier with a rifle but no bullets. This is essentially what happens in Chronic Granulomatous Disease (CGD). Neutrophils in patients with CGD can migrate to the infection and ingest the bacteria, but they lack the "ammunition" to kill them.

The defect lies in an enzyme complex called NADPH oxidase. Normally, this enzyme generates a "respiratory burst"—a rapid release of reactive oxygen species (superoxide radicals) that acts like bleach to sterilize the phagosome (the pocket inside the cell where the bacteria is trapped). In CGD, this system fails. The most common form is X-linked (affecting mostly males), caused by a mutation in the CYBB gene which codes for the gp91-phox protein.

Clinical Presentation: The Granuloma Because the neutrophils cannot kill the invaders, the immune system tries to wall them off instead. Other immune cells (macrophages and T-cells) surround the infection, forming a hard lump of tissue called a granuloma. This is why the disease is named "Granulomatous" disease.

You will typically see these patients present with:

Recurrent Abscesses: Deep skin boils or organ abscesses (liver, lungs) that are incredibly difficult to drain and heal.

Specific Pathogens: They are vulnerable to catalase-positive organisms. Bacteria like Staphylococcus aureus and fungi like Aspergillus produce an enzyme called catalase that neutralizes the tiny amount of hydrogen peroxide the patient might produce. It's a double hit to the immune system.

Gut Inflammation: Many patients develop a condition indistinguishable from Crohn's disease, caused by the immune system's frustration and over-activation in the gut lining.

Diagnosis: The Shift to DHR In the past, we used the Nitroblue Tetrazolium (NBT) slide test—a messy, subjective test where a drop of blood would turn blue if the cells worked. In 2026, the NBT test is considered obsolete.

The gold standard is the Dihydrorhodamine (DHR) Oxidation Assay. This uses flow cytometry (a laser-based cell counter).

How it works: We stimulate the neutrophils. If they produce the respiratory burst, the DHR dye glows bright green (fluoresces).

The Result: In CGD patients, there is no glow. The histogram remains flat. This test is faster, more accurate, and can even identify female carriers of the X-linked form (who will show a "mosaic" pattern of some working and some broken cells).

Management in 2026: The Era of Gene Editing The management of CGD has undergone a revolution.

Prophylaxis (The Shield): Patients are on lifelong antibiotics (usually Trimethoprim-Sulfamethoxazole) and antifungals (Itraconazole) to prevent infection.

The Cure (HSCT): Hematopoietic Stem Cell Transplantation (bone marrow transplant) remains the standard cure, but it carries risks like Graft-versus-Host Disease (GvHD).

The Frontier (Gene Therapy): This is the most exciting update for our 2026 curriculum. Following the success of trials in 2024 (such as the p47-CGD trials at Great Ormond Street), autologous gene therapy is becoming a viable option for those without a donor. This involves taking the patient's own stem cells, using a viral vector to insert a working copy of the gene, and putting them back. Even newer "Base Editing" techniques are now entering clinical practice, fixing the typo in the DNA without even cutting the double helix.

Congenital Neutropenias

If CGD is a soldier with no bullets, Congenital Neutropenia is an army with no soldiers. These are disorders where the bone marrow simply fails to produce enough mature neutrophils.

Kostmann Syndrome (Severe Congenital Neutropenia) This is the classic, severe form. Infants present almost immediately after birth with fever, umbilical cord infections, and dangerously low neutrophil counts (often near zero).

Genetics: It is often caused by mutations in the ELANE gene (neutrophil elastase) or HAX1.

The HAX1 Connection: Interestingly, the HAX1 mutation can also affect the brain, leading to neurological issues or cognitive delay, linking the immune system directly to the nervous system.

Cyclic Neutropenia This condition is mysterious and rhythmic. Patients have normal neutrophil counts most of the time, but every 21 days (roughly), their counts drop to near zero for a few days. During this "nadir" (low point), they get mouth ulcers, fevers, and infections. Then, they recover. It is often a milder version of the ELANE mutation found in Kostmann syndrome.

Management: The G-CSF Balance The mainstay of treatment is G-CSF (Granulocyte Colony-Stimulating Factor). This is a synthetic hormone that screams at the bone marrow to produce more cells.

The Success: It keeps most children alive and infection-free.

The Risk: We now know that pushing the bone marrow this hard, for years, carries a price. High doses of G-CSF over long periods can stress the marrow cells, increasing the risk of the cells transforming into leukemia (MDS/AML). In 2026, we carefully balance the dose: just enough to prevent infection, but not enough to "burn out" the marrow.

Module 11.2: Complement Deficiencies
The Bridge Between Worlds

The Complement System is a cascade of proteins (C1 through C9) that circulate in your blood like dormant landmines. When triggered, they explode into action, punching holes in bacteria and flagging them for destruction. It bridges the gap between the "dumb" innate immune system and the "smart" adaptive immune system.

When this system breaks, the type of infection you get depends entirely on where the chain is broken.

Early Component Deficiencies (C1, C2, C4)

The "Lupus Link" This is one of the most fascinating concepts in immunology. You might expect an immune deficiency to cause only infections. But Early Component deficiencies (specifically C1q, C2, and C4) primarily cause Autoimmunity.

Why? One of the main jobs of C1q is to act as a "garbage man." Every day, your body cells die and break down. C1q binds to this cellular trash (apoptotic debris) and helps clear it away quietly.

The Failure: If you lack C1q, this cellular trash builds up. Your immune system eventually "sees" the inside of its own dead cells (DNA, histones) and attacks them. This creates auto-antibodies (like Anti-Nuclear Antibodies), leading to Systemic Lupus Erythematosus (SLE).

The Stat: Nearly 90% of patients with a complete C1q deficiency will develop Lupus. It is the strongest genetic link to Lupus known in medicine.

Infection Risk Besides Lupus, these patients struggle with Encapsulated Bacteria (like Streptococcus pneumoniae). The capsule around these bugs makes them slippery; without the "sticky" complement proteins (C3b) coating them (opsonization), phagocytes can't grab them.

Late Component Deficiencies (C5-C9)

The Terminal Pathway The end goal of the complement cascade is to form the Membrane Attack Complex (MAC). This is a literal tube made of proteins (C5 through C9) that drills a hole into the surface of a bacterium, causing it to pop.

The Neisseria Specialist Most bacteria are weak enough to be killed by simple phagocytosis. But Neisseria species (the bugs that cause Meningitis and Gonorrhea) have thick cell walls that are very resistant. They require the MAC drill to be destroyed.

The Clinical Picture: If a patient comes to you with a second or third episode of Meningococcal Meningitis, you must test their Late Complement pathway (CH50 test). They are specifically vulnerable to this one family of bacteria. They handle other infections (flu, staph, strep) just fine, but Neisseria is their kryptonite.

Management and Therapeutics in 2026

Vaccination is Key For complement-deficient patients, vaccines are life-saving. We cannot repair the missing protein, so we must arm the adaptive immune system (antibodies) to compensate.

The Regimen: Patients must receive the MenACWY and MenB vaccines (for Meningitis) and the Pneumococcal vaccines. In 2026, we also emphasize boosters more frequently than the general population because their memory response needs to be robust to bypass the complement defect.

The New Era of Complement Inhibitors While this module focuses on deficiency, we must acknowledge a major 2026 therapeutic shift: treating complement excess. Disorders like C3 Glomerulopathy (C3G) or Paroxysmal Nocturnal Hemoglobinuria (PNH) are caused by too much complement activity.

New Drugs: We now have precise inhibitors like Pegcetacoplan (a C3 inhibitor) and Iptacopan (a Factor B inhibitor, approved in 2024/2025). These drugs surgically stop the cascade at specific points. While they save kidneys and red blood cells, they artificially create a "complement deficiency" in the patient.

The Irony: By treating one disease, we give the patient the same susceptibility to infection as the genetic disorders we just discussed. Therefore, a patient on Iptacopan needs the same vaccination protocol as a patient born with a C5 deficiency.

11.3 Autoimmune Lymphoproliferative Syndrome (ALPS)

1. The Core Defect: A Broken "Off Switch"

Imagine an army that recruits soldiers for a battle. Once the battle is won, those soldiers must be dismissed to save resources. In the immune system, this dismissal is called apoptosis (programmed cell death).

ALPS is caused by a genetic failure in this dismissal process.

The Pathway: The Fas/FasL pathway is the primary "death signal" for lymphocytes. When a T-cell or B-cell is no longer needed, the Fas receptor (CD95) on its surface binds to the Fas Ligand (FasL).

The Result: This binding triggers a cascade of enzymes called caspases (specifically Caspase 8 and 10), which dismantle the cell from the inside.

The Defect: In ALPS, a mutation prevents this signal. The lymphocytes do not die. They accumulate.

2026 Update: While the FAS gene mutation remains the most common cause (approx. 70% of cases), recent 2025 genetic panels have expanded to include 33 genes. We now know that variants in CASP10 and FASLG can produce milder phenotypes, while the specific FAS:c. 748C > T variant is associated with severe, early-onset disease.

2. Clinical Presentation: The Triad

Trainees must learn to spot the "ALPS Triad." If you see a child with these three features, you must investigate for ALPS.

A. Chronic Non-Malignant Lymphoproliferation

This is the most visible sign. The body is physically stuffed with excess lymphocytes.

Lymphadenopathy: Swollen lymph nodes that are often massive, firm, and non-tender. They do not shrink with antibiotics.

Splenomegaly: The spleen can become enormous (hypersplenism). It traps platelets and red blood cells, worsening blood counts.

Hepatomegaly: Enlarged liver is common.

Clinical Example: A 4-year-old boy presents with "lumps in his neck" that have been there for six months. His mother notes his belly looks swollen. On exam, you feel multiple cervical and axillary nodes the size of golf balls. The spleen is palpable 5 cm below the costal margin. He has no fever and looks well otherwise. This is the classic "healthy-looking" child with ALPS.

B. Autoimmune Cytopenias

The accumulated lymphocytes are not just taking up space; they are confused. They often attack the body's own blood cells.

Autoimmune Hemolytic Anemia (AIHA): Destruction of red blood cells.

Immune Thrombocytopenia (ITP): Destruction of platelets.

Neutropenia: Destruction of neutrophils.

Evans Syndrome: The combination of AIHA and ITP. This is a huge red flag. 40% of children with Evans Syndrome actually have ALPS.

C. Lymphoma Risk

Because the cells do not die, they live long enough to acquire bad mutations. Patients have a significantly higher risk of developing Non-Hodgkin Lymphoma and Hodgkin Lymphoma. Surveillance is critical.

3. Diagnostic Workup: The 2026 Standard

We no longer rely on guesswork. The 2026 diagnostic criteria utilize highly specific biomarkers.

The Hallmark Cell: Double-Negative T-Cells (DNTs)

This is the single most important test.

Normal T-cells are either CD4+ (helpers) or CD8+ (killers).

In ALPS, the cells lose both markers but keep their T-cell receptor (TCR).

Finding: Flow cytometry shows >1.5% (often >5%) TCR αβ+ CD4- CD8- T cells. These are the "zombie" cells that failed to die.

The Biomarker Panel

If you suspect ALPS, order these four serum markers. They are highly sensitive when combined:

Vitamin B12: Paradoxically elevated (often >1500 pg/mL) without supplementation. The DNTs act as a "sponge" for B12.

Soluble Fas Ligand (sFasL): Extremely high. The body screams "DIE!" (by pumping out Fas Ligand), but the cells don't listen.

Interleukin-10 (IL-10): Elevated.

Interleukin-18 (IL-18): Elevated.

2026 Diagnostic Pearl: If a patient has chronic lymphadenopathy + elevated Vitamin B12 + elevated DNTs, the diagnosis is ALPS until proven otherwise. You can often start treatment before the genetic sequencing comes back.

4. Management: The Sirolimus Era

The management of ALPS has been revolutionized. We have moved away from chronic steroids.

First-Line: Sirolimus (Rapamycin)

Sirolimus is an mTOR inhibitor. It targets the specific metabolic pathway that ALPS cells use to survive.

Effect: It causes the lymph nodes and spleen to shrink dramatically, often within 1-3 months. It also controls the cytopenias.

Protocol: Start at 2-3 $mg/m^2/day$. Monitor trough levels (target 5-10 ng/mL).

Why it wins: Unlike steroids, it doesn't stunt growth or cause Cushing's syndrome. Unlike chemotherapy, it preserves fertility.

2026 Caution: Long-term Sirolimus use requires monitoring for hyperlipidemia and mouth sores (aphthous ulcers).

Second-Line: Mycophenolate Mofetil (MMF)

Used if Sirolimus is not tolerated. It is good for cytopenias but less effective for shrinking the large lymph nodes/spleen.
What to Avoid:

Splenectomy: In the past, doctors removed the spleen to fix low platelets. This is now contraindicated. Removing the spleen in ALPS drastically increases the risk of fatal sepsis because the rest of the immune system is already slightly compromised. Avoid taking the spleen out unless absolutely necessary.

11.4 Autoinflammatory Syndromes (Periodic Fevers)

We now shift from the "adaptive" immune system to the "innate" immune system.

These are not autoimmune diseases. There are no antibodies. There are no T-cells attacking tissues. Instead, these are disorders of danger sensing. The body thinks it is infected when it is not. The innate immune system (neutrophils, macrophages) launches a massive inflammatory attack (fever, rash, pain) for no reason.

We will cover the three major "monogenic" fever syndromes.

1. Familial Mediterranean Fever (FMF)

This is the most common periodic fever syndrome. It classically affects Jewish, Armenian, Turkish, and Arab populations.

The Defect: Mutation in the MEFV gene.

The Protein: Pyrin. Normally, Pyrin sits inside neutrophils and keeps inflammation in check. The mutation makes Pyrin unstable. It "unlocks" the inflammasome too easily.

The Cytokine: Massive release of Interleukin-1 (IL-1).

Clinical Presentation

Attacks: Short and sharp. They last 1 to 3 days.

Fever: High grade (>39°C).

Serositis: Inflammation of the linings.

Peritoneum: Severe abdominal pain (often mimics appendicitis).

Pleura: Chest pain (pleurisy).

Synovium: Arthritis (swollen knee or ankle).

Skin: Erysipelas-like erythema (a red, hot rash on the shin or foot).

Clinical Example: A 20-year-old Turkish man comes to the ER with 10/10 abdominal pain and fever. He has had 5 similar episodes this year. He has an appendectomy scar, but the surgeons found a normal appendix. This history of "sterile peritonitis" is classic FMF.

The Major Danger: Amyloidosis

If FMF is untreated, the constant inflammation produces a protein called Serum Amyloid A (SAA). This protein clumps together and clogs the kidneys, leading to renal failure (Nephrotic Syndrome).
Management

- Colchicine (The Gold Standard):
    - It is not a painkiller; it is a preventative.
    - It stabilizes the neutrophil skeleton so Pyrin doesn't misfire.
    - 2026 Guideline: Dosing is strictly weight-based. Compliance is key. Missing even one dose can trigger an attack.
- Colchicine Resistance:
    - About 5-10% of patients do not respond to Colchicine.
    - Treatment: We switch to IL-1 Blockers.
        - Anakinra: Daily injection (short-acting).
        - Canakinumab: Monthly injection (long-acting). This is highly effective for resistant FMF.

2. TNF Receptor-Associated Periodic Syndrome (TRAPS)

This is the longest-duration fever syndrome.

- The Defect: Mutation in TNFRSF1A gene.

The Mechanism: The receptor for TNF (Tumor Necrosis Factor) usually sits on the cell surface. When it's done working, it should be shed or internalized. In TRAPS, the receptor gets "stuck" open or misfolds inside the cell, causing constant stress and inflammation.

Clinical Presentation

Attacks: Long. They last 1 to 3 weeks (much longer than FMF).

Fever: High and persistent.

Eyes: Periorbital edema (puffiness around the eyes) is a distinctive sign.

Muscle: Severe myalgia (muscle pain) that moves down the limbs (migratory myalgia).

Skin: Migratory red rash that is warm to the touch.

Clinical Example: A 35-year-old woman presents with fevers that last 14 days. During these episodes, her eyes swell shut, and she has deep muscle pain in her thighs. Her father had similar "rheumatism." The long duration and eye swelling point to TRAPS.

Management

First Line: Corticosteroids (Prednisolone) work well to stop an attack, but long-term use is toxic.

Targeted Therapy: IL-1 Inhibitors (Canakinumab) are now the standard of care for maintenance.

What NOT to use: Interestingly, drugs that block TNF (like Etanercept) have had mixed/poor results, despite the disease being a TNF receptor defect. IL-1 blockade is superior.

2026 Update: Newer agents like Rilonacept (an IL-1 trap) have shown success in patients who fail Canakinumab, especially those with recurrent pericarditis.

3. Mevalonate Kinase Deficiency (MKD)

Also known as Hyper-IgD Syndrome (HIDS).

This is a metabolic autoinflammatory disease.

The Defect: Mutation in the MVK gene.

The Pathway: The mevalonate pathway produces cholesterol. The block leads to a shortage of anti-inflammatory molecules and an excess of pro-inflammatory ones.

The Trigger: Attacks are often triggered by vaccinations or mild viral infections.

Clinical Presentation

Attacks: Last 3 to 7 days.

Gastrointestinal: Vomiting, diarrhea, and abdominal pain are very prominent.

Lymph Nodes: Cervical lymphadenopathy (swollen neck nodes) during fever.

Skin: Diverse rashes (urticaria, maculopapular).

Unique Symptom: Aphthous ulcers (canker sores) in the mouth and genital region are very common.

Clinical Example: A 6-month-old infant spikes a 40°C fever 12 hours after receiving routine vaccinations. The baby vomits repeatedly and develops swollen glands in the neck. Genetic testing reveals MVK mutations.

Management

Acute Attacks: NSAIDs or short-course steroids.

Maintenance: Canakinumab is the only FDA/EMA-approved biologic that reliably controls the frequency of attacks.

2026 Data: The RELIANCE registry (published late 2025) confirmed the long-term safety of Canakinumab in MKD, showing it prevents the severe "failure to thrive" seen in untreated children.

Summary Table: The Periodic Fevers

Feature	FMF	TRAPS	MKD (HIDS)
Gene	MEFV	TNFRSF1A	MVK
Attack Duration	Short (1-3 days)	Long (1-3 weeks)	Medium (3-7 days)
Key Sign	Sterile Peritonitis (Acute Abdomen)	Periorbital Edema (Puffy Eyes)	Triggered by Vaccines; Mouth Ulcers
Mechanism	Pyrin / IL-1 excess	TNF Receptor defect	Metabolic / IL-1 excess
Treatment	Colchicine	IL-1 Blockers (Canakinumab)	IL-1 Blockers (Canakinumab)

Secondary Immunodeficiency and Immunoglobulin Stewardship

12.1 Iatrogenic Immunodeficiency: The Cost of Cure

Iatrogenic (doctor-induced) immunodeficiency is the most common form of immune dysfunction you will encounter in adult practice. It is predictable, dose-dependent, and often permanent.

1. B-Cell Depleting Therapies: The "Silent" Aplasia

Monoclonal antibodies targeting CD20 (Rituximab, Ocrelizumab, Ofatumumab) have revolutionized the treatment of Rheumatoid Arthritis (RA), Multiple Sclerosis (MS), and vasculitis. By lysing CD20+ B-cells, these drugs halt the production of pathogenic autoantibodies.

However, CD20 is not just on "bad" B-cells. It is on all mature B-cells.

The Mechanism of Deficit: When you administer Rituximab, you induce a state of B-cell aplasia. The peripheral B-cell count drops to zero. While plasma cells (which produce antibodies) do not express CD20 and are initially spared, they eventually die off. Without a B-cell pool to replenish them, antibody levels (IgG, IgM, IgA) begin a slow, inexorable decline. This is "hypogammaglobulinemia by attrition."

Clinical Pearl: In 2026, we now understand that Ocrelizumab (used in MS) carries a cumulative risk. The drop in IgG may not be clinically apparent for the first two years, but by year five, a significant cohort of patients drops below the protective threshold of 4g/L.

The Infection Profile: Patients do not typically present with opportunistic infections like Pneumocystis (unless on steroids). Instead, they present with:

Sino-pulmonary infections: Recurrent bacterial pneumonia (Streptococcus pneumoniae, Haemophilus influenzae).

Chronic Enteroviral Meningoencephalitis: A rare but devastating complication where the body cannot clear common enteroviruses due to a lack of antibodies.

The Vaccine Void: The most critical 2026 update regarding anti-CD20 therapy involves vaccination. B-cell depleted patients cannot mount a humoral response to new antigens. If you vaccinate a patient on Rituximab against a novel influenza strain or a SARS-CoV-2 variant, they will likely produce zero antibodies. T-cell responses may remain, preventing death, but sterilizing immunity is lost.

Example: Consider a 45-year-old woman with RA treated with Rituximab. She receives her annual flu shot. Three months later, she is hospitalized with severe Influenza A. Her "failure" to respond to the vaccine was not a biological anomaly; it was a predicted pharmacological outcome of her therapy.

2. CAR-T Cell Therapy: Engineering Immunity

Chimeric Antigen Receptor T-cell (CAR-T) therapy involves harvesting a patient's T-cells, genetically reprogramming them to hunt CD19+ or BCMA+ cells, and re-infusing them.

Two Phases of Risk:

The Storm (Days 0–30): The immediate risk is Cytokine Release Syndrome (CRS). The immune system goes into overdrive, releasing IL-6 and TNF-alpha. This mimics severe sepsis. We treat this with Tocilizumab (an IL-6 blocker), which itself causes a transient immunodeficiency, masking fever and CRP rise.

The Long Winter (Months 1–Indefinite): The CAR-T cells are "living drugs." They persist in the body, patrolling for malignancy. As long as they persist, they kill all B-cells. This results in profound, sustained B-cell aplasia.

2026 Perspective - The "Reset": Recent EULAR 2025 and ASH 2025 data have highlighted the use of CAR-T in severe autoimmune diseases (like refractory Lupus). The goal here is an "immune reset." Interestingly, in autoimmune cohorts, B-cells may eventually recover without the disease returning. However, in cancer cohorts, permanent aplasia is often the goal to prevent relapse.

Management: Post-CAR-T patients often require Immunoglobulin Replacement Therapy (IgRT) indefinitely if their IgG levels fall and infection rates rise. They also require prophylaxis against Pneumocystis jirovecii (PJP) and Herpes Zoster (Shingles) until their CD4 count recovers, which can lag months behind clinical recovery.

3. Novel Small Molecules: The Signal Blockers

We have moved beyond broad chemotherapy to "targeted" small molecules. These drugs block specific intracellular pathways.

BTK Inhibitors (Ibrutinib, Zanubrutinib, Pirtobrutinib): Used in CLL and lymphoma. Bruton's Tyrosine Kinase (BTK) is essential for B-cell maturation. Blocking it stops the cancer but creates functional antibody deficiency.

Update: The 2026 landscape includes "BTK Degraders" (like Bexobrutideg). These destroy the protein entirely.

While effective against resistant tumors, the depth of immune suppression may be more profound.

Fungal Signal: Unlike pure antibody deficiency, BTK inhibitors have a unique signal for Invasive Aspergillosis, likely because BTK plays a role in macrophage function, not just B-cells.

JAK Inhibitors (Tofacitinib, Upadacitinib): Used in RA, eczema, and alopecia. These block the "telephone lines" of the immune system (cytokine signaling).

The Shingles Signal: The most consistent risk is Herpes Zoster reactivation. JAK inhibitors block the interferon signaling required to keep viral latency in check.

4. The ACI Physician's Role: The "Shield"

Your role is not to stop the therapy—the therapy is keeping the cancer or autoimmunity at bay. Your role is to build a shield around the patient.

The "ACI Protocol" for Iatrogenic Patients:

Baseline Risk Stratification: Measure IgG, IgA, IgM, and specific antibody titers (Tetanus, Pneumococcus) before starting therapy (the "Pre-Rituximab Checklist").

Vaccination Window: Vaccinate at least 4 weeks before B-cell depletion. If the patient is already depleted, vaccination is often deferred until B-cells reconstitute (CD19 > 1%).

Surveillance: Monitor IgG levels every 3–6 months.

Intervention:

Antibiotic Prophylaxis: Azithromycin 250mg 3x/week is the first line for recurrent respiratory infections.

Ig Replacement: Only if antibiotic prophylaxis fails (see Section 12.2).

12.2 Malignancy-Associated Immunodeficiency: The "Immune Paresis"

In hematological malignancies, the immune system is doubly hit: first by the cancer itself, and second by the treatment.

The Concept of "Immune Paresis"

In Chronic Lymphocytic Leukemia (CLL) and Multiple Myeloma (MM), the bone marrow is hijacked.

In Myeloma: The malignant plasma cells crowd out the healthy plasma cells. They produce a monoclonal protein (M-spike) that is useless for fighting infection, while the production of functional polyclonal immunoglobulins (IgG, IgA, IgM) is suppressed. This suppression of healthy antibody production is called "immune paresis."

In CLL: The leukemic cells secrete immunosuppressive cytokines (like TGF-beta/IL-10) that inhibit the function of normal T-cells and B-cells.

The Consequence: Infection is the leading cause of death in CLL and Myeloma. These patients are functionally hypogammaglobulinemic even before they receive a single dose of chemotherapy.

The "LLMP" Criteria for Management

Managing this deficiency is expensive and burdensome. We cannot give Immunoglobulin Replacement Therapy (IgRT) to everyone with a low number. We use the LLMP Criteria (Lymphoma, Leukemia, Myeloma Protocols) to determine eligibility.

The LLMP Decision Triad: To qualify for IgRT (IVIG or SCIG) in 2026, a patient typically must meet three strict criteria. This ensures stewardship of the plasma supply (a finite human resource).

Quantitative Failure:

Serum IgG < 4 g/L (excluding the paraprotein/M-spike).

Note: If IgG is > 4g/L but < Lower Limit of Normal, they may still qualify if they have "Functional Antibody Deficiency" (failure to respond to test vaccination).

Clinical Failure:

History of severe, recurrent, or persistent bacterial infections.

"Severe" = Requires hospitalization or IV antibiotics.

"Recurrent" = >3 infections per year.

Therapeutic Failure (The "Antibiotic Trial"):

The patient must have failed a trial of continuous prophylactic antibiotics (e.g., Azithromycin or Co-trimoxazole for 3 months).

Rationale: Antibiotics are cheap, oral, and effective for many. IgRT is expensive, biological, and requires infusions. If Azithromycin stops the pneumonia, IgRT is not indicated.

Example: A 68-year-old male with CLL has an IgG of 3.2 g/L. He gets one sinus infection a year. Action: Do not treat with IgRT. Observation only.

Contrast: The same male has an IgG of 3.2 g/L. He has had three hospital admissions for pneumonia this year despite taking prophylactic Azithromycin. Action: Initiate IgRT immediately. He meets the LLMP criteria (Low IgG + Clinical Failure + Antibiotic Failure).

Balancing Burden vs. Benefit

The ACI physician must weigh the "Infection Burden" against the "Therapy Burden."

Therapy Burden: IVIG requires hospital visits every 3–4 weeks. SCIG (Subcutaneous) allows home therapy but requires the patient to insert needles into their abdomen weekly. For a frail Myeloma patient with bone pain, this is physically demanding.

Infection Burden: Repeated hospitalizations degrade quality of life and interrupt cancer treatment (chemotherapy must be paused during active infection).

The 2026 Standard of Care: We now favor SCIG (Subcutaneous Ig) for these patients. It maintains steady-state IgG levels (no "wear-off" effect at the end of the month) and keeps immunocompromised patients out of the hospital environment where nosocomial infections lurk.

12.3 Immunoglobulin Replacement Therapy (IgRT): Modalities & Mechanics

As a trainee, your goal is not just to prescribe Ig. Your goal is to match the mode of delivery to the life of the patient. Let's break down the two main contenders: IVIG and SCIG.

1. The Great Debate: IVIG versus SCIG

Think of these two modalities as two different ways to charge a battery.

IVIG (Intravenous Immunoglobulin): The "Supercharger"

How it works: You infuse a large dose directly into the vein every 3 or 4 weeks.

The Experience: The patient comes to the hospital (or has a nurse visit). They sit for 2–4 hours hooked up to a drip.

The "Sawtooth" Pattern: This is critical. IVIG causes a massive spike in IgG levels immediately after infusion (the peak). Then, the levels drop rapidly over the next few weeks until they hit rock bottom (the trough) right before the next dose.

Side Effects: Because of that massive initial spike, patients often feel systemic side effects. Headache. Fever. Fatigue. It's a "boom and bust" cycle.

Who is it for?

Example: Meet Sarah. She is 24 and unreliable with daily tasks. She forgets pills. She prefers to come to the hospital once a month, get her "fill," and forget about it for 30 days. IVIG suits her lifestyle.

SCIG (Subcutaneous Immunoglobulin): The "Trickle Charger"

How it works: The patient infuses a smaller dose under the skin (usually the stomach or thigh) once a week, or even daily. No veins are needed.

The Experience: This is done at home. It takes about 1 hour. Patients can watch TV or read while it happens.

The "Steady State": There are no massive peaks or deep troughs. The IgG levels stay flat and stable.

Side Effects: Systemic side effects (headaches) are rare because there is no spike. The main issue is local swelling or redness at the injection site (we call this a "bee sting" reaction), but it usually fades.

Who is it for?

Example: Meet David. He is a busy architect with difficult veins (venous access issues). He travels for work. He cannot be tied to a hospital schedule. He packs his SCIG pump in his suitcase and infuses in his hotel room. SCIG gives him freedom.

2. Pharmacokinetics: Mastering the "Trough"

In 2026, we do not guess doses. We calculate them.

The Concept of the "Trough" The "trough level" is the lowest amount of IgG in the patient's blood right before their next infusion. If the trough is too low, the patient is unprotected for the last few days of their cycle. This is when "breakthrough infections" happen.

The Goal: We used to aim for a generic number (e.g., 6 g/L). Now, we aim for a "biological trough." This means we push the dose up until the patient stops getting infections. For a patient with severe lung damage (bronchiectasis), a trough of 6 g/L is not enough; they might need 9 g/L or 10 g/L to stay healthy.

Visualizing the Difference:

IVIG: Imagine filling a bathtub to the brim (Peak) and then pulling the plug. The water drains out slowly. You have to refill it before it's empty (Trough).

SCIG: Imagine a bathtub with the drain open, but the tap is constantly running at a slow, steady trickle. The water level never changes.

3. Specialty CiP 5: Home Therapy Training

Training a patient to treat themselves is a core competency (Specialty CiP 5). You are not just a doctor here; you are a teacher.

The Process: It is not instant. It takes 4 to 6 weeks of training sessions.

The Curriculum: You must teach them to:

Inspect the product: Is the liquid clear? Is it expired?

Sterile technique: Wash hands. Clean the skin. Avoid infection.

Troubleshooting: What if the pump alarm beeps? What if there is blood in the tubing?

Anaphylaxis drill: It is rare, but patients must know how to use an adrenaline auto-injector if they have a severe reaction.

The Benefit: Home therapy saves the hospital money (fewer bed days) and gives the patient control.

12.4 Stewardship and Commissioning: The "Gatekeepers"

In 2026, plasma supply is fragile. We rely on donations from a few key countries (mostly the USA). If that supply chain breaks, patients die. Therefore, we practice Stewardship. You cannot just prescribe Ig because you "think it might help." You must prove it is necessary.

1. The Traffic Light System: Red, Blue, and Grey

To manage demand, we categorize diseases by color. You must memorize these categories to pass the IAP (Immunoglobulin Assessment Panel).

Red Indications (Critical):

Definition: Life-threatening. Treatment is mandatory. No debate.

Example: A baby with Kawasaki Disease. Without Ig, they could develop heart aneurysms.

Example: Primary Immunodeficiency (PID) where the body makes no antibodies at all.

Blue Indications (Necessary but Negotiable):

Definition: There is good evidence that Ig works, but there might be other drugs (like steroids or Rituximab) that should be tried first.

Example: ITP (Immune Thrombocytopenia). Ig raises the platelet count, but steroids are cheaper and often work just as well. You only use Ig if steroids fail or if surgery is urgent.

Grey Indications (The Danger Zone):

Definition: These are rare, immune-mediated diseases where the evidence is weak. Maybe it works, maybe it doesn't.

The Rule: You cannot just prescribe for a Grey indication. You must apply to the panel. You must set a "stop date." If the patient does not improve after 3 months, you must stop the therapy.

Example: Chronic Fatigue Syndrome typically falls here (or is often "Black" - not recommended).

Example: Secondary Antibody Deficiency (e.g., after cancer treatment). This is the biggest area of debate in 2026.

2. The IAP: The Immunoglobulin Assessment Panel

Every hospital (or region) has an IAP. This is a group of experts—immunologists, haematologists, pharmacists—who act as the gatekeepers.

The Process:

You see a patient. You want to give Ig.

You fill out a request form. You must state the "Indication Color" (Red, Blue, Grey).

If it is Blue or Grey, the IAP reviews it. They ask: "Have you tried cheaper drugs? Is this dose correct?"

Approval: If approved, funding is released for a specific time (e.g., 6 months).

The "Pay-for-Performance" Twist: The IAP demands data. If you do not record the patient's trough levels and infection rates in the national database, the funding gets cut. This ensures we aren't wasting "liquid gold" on patients who aren't getting better.

3. Demand Management Plan

What happens if there is a global shortage? (This happened in 2019, 2022, and again recently). We move to a Demand Management Plan.

Step 1: Protect the Red indications (the babies, the severe PID cases).

Step 2: Cut the Grey indications. Stop therapy for anyone where the benefit is "maybe."

Step 3: Reduce doses. Patients on Blue indications might have their dose cut by 10% or 20% to stretch the supply.

The Reality: This is painful. You have to look a patient in the eye and say, "I know this medicine helps you feel energetic, but we have to save it for someone who will die without it." This is the hardest part of stewardship.

Autoimmunity, Vasculitis, and Systemic Inflammation

13.1 Systemic Lupus Erythematosus (SLE) and Connective Tissue Diseases (CTDs)

Systemic Lupus Erythematosus (SLE) remains the prototype of systemic autoimmunity. It is a disease of "loss of tolerance," where the body's immune system creates a broad spectrum of antibodies against its own nuclear material.

A. The Autoantibody Profile: The "Fingerprint" of Disease

For the ACI physician, the autoantibody profile is not just a checklist; it is a prognostic map. We do not treat antibodies, we treat patients—but the antibodies tell us where the disease might strike next.

1. Anti-Nuclear Antibody (ANA): The Gatekeeper The ANA remains the entry-level screening test. By 2026 standards, we emphasize that a positive ANA is necessary but not sufficient for an SLE diagnosis.

Sensitivity: Extremely high (>98%). A negative ANA essentially rules out SLE (with rare exceptions).

Specificity: Low. Positive ANAs are found in healthy individuals, thyroid disease, and infections.

Patterns Matter: We look for the "Homogeneous" or "Speckled" patterns on immunofluorescence. *

2. Anti-dsDNA (Double-Stranded DNA): The Nephritis Marker

Significance: This is highly specific for SLE. It is one of the few antibodies that fluctuates with disease activity.

Clinical Pearl: If anti-dsDNA levels rise, the risk of a "flare"—specifically Lupus Nephritis (kidney inflammation)—increases. In 2026 protocols, a rising titer often triggers preemptive urinalysis monitoring.

3. Anti-Sm (Smith): The Specificity King

Significance: Anti-Sm is the most specific antibody for SLE. If a patient has this, they almost certainly have Lupus.

Sensitivity: Low (only found in ~30% of patients). Its absence does not rule out the disease.

4. Anti-Ro (SS-A) and Anti-La (SS-B): The Cross-Over Agents
These antibodies are the bridge between Lupus and Sjogren's Syndrome.

Neonatal Risk: In pregnant women, Anti-Ro/La can cross the placenta and cause Neonatal Lupus, leading to a congenital heart block. This is a critical counseling point.

Photosensitivity: Patients with these antibodies are often exquisitely sensitive to sunlight, developing subacute cutaneous lupus rashes.

B. Clinical Correlations: From Skin to Kidney

Lupus Nephritis This is the major cause of morbidity. Immune complexes (clumps of antibody and antigen) get stuck in the delicate filters of the kidney (glomeruli).

The "Silent" Killer: Early nephritis has no symptoms. It is detected only by protein or blood in the urine.

2026 Management Shift: We are seeing a move toward early "multitarget therapy"—combining biologic agents (like belimumab) with standard immunosuppression to preserve kidney function earlier.

Cutaneous (Skin) Lupus

Malar Rash: The classic "butterfly rash" across the cheeks, sparing the nasolabial folds (the lines from nose to mouth).

Discoid Lupus: These are scarring, coin-shaped lesions that can lead to permanent hair loss (alopecia). *

C. Overlap Syndromes: When Diseases Collide

Autoimmune diseases rarely read the textbooks; they often blend together.

1. Mixed Connective Tissue Disease (MCTD) Think of MCTD as a "salad" of symptoms: some Lupus, some Scleroderma (thick skin), and some Myositis (muscle inflammation).

The Hallmark: The defining feature is a very high titer of Anti-U1-RNP antibody.

The Danger: Unlike pure Lupus, MCTD carries a specific high risk for Pulmonary Arterial Hypertension (PAH), which requires vigilant screening.

2. Sjogren's Syndrome Often secondary to SLE, this involves the destruction of moisture-producing glands.

Symptoms: Sicca symptoms (dry eyes, dry mouth).

Antibodies: Anti-Ro (SSA) and Anti-La (SSB).

The Lymphoma Risk: A critical 2026 update is the heightened awareness that Sjogren's patients have a significantly increased risk of B-cell lymphoma. Persistent swollen glands must be biopsied.

D. 2026 Spotlight: CAR-T Cell Therapy in SLE

Perhaps the most exciting development in this module is the maturation of Chimeric Antigen Receptor (CAR) T-cell therapy. Originally designed for cancer, this "living drug" is now used for refractory SLE.

Mechanism: We harvest the patient's T-cells, engineer them to recognize CD19 (a protein on B-cells), and infuse them back. These "hunter" T-cells wipe out the B-cells that produce the bad antibodies.

The Result: Early data from 2024-2025 trials showed "drug-free remission"—meaning patients could stop all steroids and immunosuppressants. By 2026, this is becoming a viable option for severe, life-threatening Lupus that has failed standard therapy.

13.2 Systemic Vasculitis

Systemic vasculitis is the inflammation of blood vessel walls. It is categorized by the size of the vessel involved: Large, Medium, or Small.
A. ANCA-Associated Vasculitis (AAV)

The small-vessel vasculitides are dominated by the presence of Anti-Neutrophil Cytoplasmic Antibodies (ANCA). These antibodies attack neutrophils (white blood cells), causing them to degranulate and damage vessel walls.

1. The Two Main Patterns (Immunofluorescence)

c-ANCA (Cytoplasmic): The glow is throughout the neutrophil. This strongly correlates with the antigen PR3 (Proteinase 3).

p-ANCA (Perinuclear): The glow is around the nucleus. This strongly correlates with the antigen MPO (Myeloperoxidase). *

2. The Three Diseases

Disease	Associated ANCA	Key Clinical Features
Granulomatosis with Polyangiitis (GPA)	c-ANCA (PR3)	"Head and Kidney": Sinusitis, saddle-nose deformity, cavitating lung nodules, and kidney failure. Granulomas are seen on biopsy.
Microscopic Polyangiitis (MPA)	p-ANCA (MPO)	"Kidney and Lung": Similar to GPA but without the granulomas or severe sinus involvement. Pulmonary hemorrhage is a risk.
Eosinophilic Granulomatosis with Polyangiitis (EGPA)	p-ANCA (MPO)	"Asthma and Eosinophils": Patients almost always have adult-onset asthma and high eosinophil counts. Can affect the heart.

3. 2026 Management Updates

Avacopan: As of the 2025 guidelines, Avacopan (a complement C5a receptor inhibitor) has largely replaced high-dose steroids for induction in many centers. It reduces the toxicity associated with long-term prednisone use.

Mepolizumab: For EGPA, this anti-IL-5 biologic is now the gold standard for controlling the eosinophilic component of the disease.

B. Large Vessel Vasculitis

Giant Cell Arteritis (GCA)

Target: The temporal arteries (temples) and aorta.

Risk: Sudden, permanent blindness if the ophthalmic artery is blocked.

Urgency: This is a medical emergency. If suspected (headache, jaw claudication, scalp tenderness), start steroids immediately before biopsy.

C. Immune Complex Vasculitis: Cryoglobulinemia

This is a unique form of vasculitis where immunoglobulins precipitate (turn into sludge) in the cold.

1. The Types

Type I: Monoclonal IgM. Usually due to blood cancers (Multiple Myeloma).

Type II (Mixed): Monoclonal IgM + Polyclonal IgG. This is the classic "Mixed Cryoglobulinemia." 90% of cases are caused by Hepatitis C.

Type III (Mixed): Polyclonal IgM + Polyclonal IgG. Seen in autoimmune diseases like Lupus.

2. The "Melt" Phenotype Patients present with the "Meltzers Triad":

Purpura: Rash on legs.

Arthralgia: Joint pain.

Weakness.

3. The Critical Laboratory Interface: Warm Transport This is the most common reason for diagnostic failure in this module.

The Problem: Cryoglobulins precipitate below body temperature (37°C). If you draw blood and let it sit on the counter (20°C), the cryoglobulins will fall out of the serum before the lab measures it. The test will be falsely negative.

The Protocol:

Pre-warm the needle and collection tube to 37°C.

Draw the blood.

Transport the sample in a thermos or warm water bath at 37°C immediately to the lab.

Centrifuge at 37°C.

13.3 Organ-Specific Autoimmunity

This section deals with diseases where the immune system targets specific proteins within a single organ. While the damage is localized, the implications are systemic.

1. Autoimmune Thyroid Disease (AITD)

The thyroid remains the most common target of autoimmune attack.

Hashimoto's Thyroiditis This is the archetype of organ-specific destruction. T-cells infiltrate the thyroid gland. They mistake normal thyroid proteins for threats.

The Mechanism: The body produces antibodies against Thyroid Peroxidase (TPO) and Thyroglobulin (Tg). These are not just markers; they signal an active siege. The gland becomes inflamed (lymphocytic infiltration). Over time, the functional tissue is replaced by fibrosis. The thyroid slowly dies.

2026 Perspective: We now recognize a "pre-Hashimoto's" phase. In 2026, we don't just wait for TSH to rise. We monitor antibody titers in high-risk groups (like those with Type 1 Diabetes). Early intervention with selenium and immune-modulators is currently being trialed to stop the destruction before hypothyroidism sets in.

Clinical Example: A patient presents with vague fatigue. Their TSH is normal. However, TPO antibodies are sky-high. In previous years, we did nothing. Now, we recognize this as "Euthyroid Autoimmune Disease." We monitor these patients for the sudden development of goiter or other autoimmune clusters.

Graves' Disease This is the opposite of Hashimoto's. Instead of destroying the gland, the immune system hijacks it.

The Mechanism: The body creates Thyroid Stimulating Immunoglobulins (TSI). These antibodies mimic TSH. They bind to the TSH receptor and turn it "on." The switch gets stuck. The thyroid floods the body with hormone (thyrotoxicosis).

New Therapies: In 2026, we are moving away from radioactive iodine which destroys the gland. New Fc-receptor blocking agents are entering clinical use. These drugs wash the autoantibodies out of the blood without damaging the thyroid tissue itself.

2. Coeliac Disease: The Systemic Intolerance

Coeliac disease is no longer considered just a "food allergy." It is a multi-system autoimmune disorder triggered by gluten.

The Immunological Trigger Tissue Transglutaminase (tTG) is the enemy here. It is an enzyme in the gut. When gluten is eaten, tTG modifies it. The immune system sees this modified gluten-tTG complex as a virus-like threat.

The Antibodies: We test for IgA-tTG and IgA-Endomysial antibodies (EMA).

The 2026 Standard: Biopsy is still the gold standard, but "serology-based diagnosis" is now accepted for children with very high antibody levels (greater than 10x the upper limit). This saves thousands of children from invasive gastroscopy.

The "Iceberg" Concept For every symptomatic patient with diarrhea, there are seven "silent" patients. They may present only with iron deficiency anemia or osteoporosis.

Example: A young woman comes in with repeated fractures. She has no stomach pain. A savvy immunologist checks for Coeliac disease. Her gut lining is flat (villous atrophy), causing poor calcium absorption. Treating the gut fixes the bones.

3. Autoimmune Liver Disease

The liver is a master of immune tolerance. It filters blood from the gut, which is full of bacteria. It must ignore them. When this tolerance breaks, the liver destroys itself.

Primary Biliary Cholangitis (PBC)

Target: The small bile ducts.

Marker: Anti-Mitochondrial Antibodies (AMA). This is one of the most specific tests in medicine. If you have AMA, you almost certainly have PBC.

Clinical Picture: The classic patient is a middle-aged woman with intense itching (pruritus) but no rash. The bile ducts are being destroyed, causing bile acids to spill into the blood.

Autoimmune Hepatitis (AIH)

Target: The liver cells (hepatocytes) themselves.

Markers: Smooth Muscle Antibodies (SMA) and Anti-LKM (Liver Kidney Microsomal).

The Danger: This is an aggressive disease. It can progress to cirrhosis in months if untreated.

2026 Update: We have identified genetic subsets of AIH that respond poorly to steroids. We now use genetic profiling early to switch these patients to second-line agents like mycophenolate mofetil (MMF) immediately, sparing them the side effects of high-dose prednisone.

4. Pernicious Anemia

This is often forgotten. It is the autoimmune destruction of the stomach lining (atrophic gastritis).

The Mechanism The immune system attacks Parietal Cells. These cells have two jobs: make acid and make Intrinsic

Factor (IF). IF is a "taxi" for Vitamin B12. Without the taxi, B12 cannot cross the gut wall.

The Result: The patient runs out of B12. Red blood cells become huge and fragile (Megaloblastic Anemia). Nerves begin to die (neuropathy).

The Connection: In 2026, we see this often linked with thyroid disease. If a thyroid patient is tired despite normal TSH, check their B12. It is likely Pernicious Anemia.

5. Polyautoimmunity: The Clustering Effect

Autoimmunity loves company. If a patient has one disease, the risk of a second is high. We call these Autoimmune Polyglandular Syndromes (APS).

APS Type 1: A rare genetic failure (AIRE gene mutation). It appears in childhood.

Triad: Candidiasis (yeast infections), Hypoparathyroidism, Addison's disease.

APS Type 2 (Schmidt's Syndrome): The most common adult form.

Combination: Addison's disease + Thyroid disease + Type 1 Diabetes.

Course Note: In 2026, we use "predictive clustering." If a patient has Addison's disease (adrenal failure), we automatically screen for Coeliac and Thyroid antibodies annually. We do not wait for symptoms.

13.4 Autoimmune Encephalitis and Neurological Antibodies

This is the most exciting frontier in immunology today. Ten years ago, these patients were often misdiagnosed as "crazy" or "psychotic." They were sent to psychiatric wards. Today, we know their immune system is attacking their brain.

We divide these into two main categories: Cell Surface Antibodies (directly pathogenic) and Intracellular Antibodies (markers of cancer).
1. Anti-NMDA Receptor Encephalitis

This is the poster child of the field.

The Target The NMDA receptor controls memory and learning. It is the brain's main excitatory switch.

The Attack: Antibodies bind to the receptor and force it to be internalized (swallowed) by the neuron. The brain essentially runs out of switches. The hardware is fine, but the software crashes.

Clinical Progression:

Viral Prodrome: Fever, headache (looks like the flu).

Psychiatric Phase: Paranoia, hallucinations, bizarre behavior. (Often misdiagnosed as Schizophrenia).

Neurological Phase: Seizures, movement disorders (mouth movements, dyskinesia), catatonia.

Autonomic Instability: Heart rate and blood pressure fluctuate wildly.

2026 Treatment: We are faster now. We don't wait for the antibody test to come back from the lab. If the "NMDA score" is high, we start plasma exchange (PLEX) immediately. We wash the blood to remove the antibodies.

2. The Voltage-Gated Potassium Channel Complex (LGI1 and CASPR2)

These were formerly lumped together. Now we know they are distinct.

Anti-LGI1 Encephalitis

Presentation: This affects older men mostly. It causes a very specific seizure called Faciobrachial Dystonic Seizures (FBDS).

The Sign: The patient's arm and face twitch violently for just a second, dozens of times a day.

Why it matters: These seizures are a warning shot. If treated with steroids now, we prevent the massive memory loss (dementia) that follows. Anti-epileptic drugs do not work here. Only immunotherapy works.

Anti-CASPR2 Encephalitis

Presentation: This is a slower burn. It affects the peripheral nerves too.

Morvan's Syndrome: A mix of muscle twitching (neuromyotonia), insomnia (unable to sleep for days), and confusion. It is rare but unforgettable.

3. Paraneoplastic Syndromes (Intracellular Antigens)

These are different. The antibodies here (Hu, Yo, Ri) do not cause the damage directly. They are smoke signals.

The Mechanism A tumor (usually hidden) expresses a neuronal protein. The immune system attacks the tumor (good!) but then gets confused and attacks the brain (bad!).

T-Cell Mediated: The damage is done by Killer T-cells, not the antibodies. This means removing the antibodies (via plasma exchange) often fails. You must find and kill the cancer.

The "Big Three" Panels

Anti-Hu (ANNA-1): Linked to Small Cell Lung Cancer. Causes sensory neuropathy (loss of sensation) and cerebellar degeneration.

Anti-Yo (PCA-1): Linked to Ovarian or Breast Cancer. Causes rapid onset clumsiness (cerebellar ataxia). A woman who could walk fine last week is now wheelchair-bound.

Anti-Ri (ANNA-2): Linked to Breast Cancer. Causes opsoclonus-myoclonus (dancing eyes and dancing feet).

The 2026 Approach to Paraneoplastic Screening We now use "Liquid Biopsy" alongside antibody panels. We look for circulating tumor DNA in the blood. If we find Anti-Yo, we scan the patient from head to toe. If the scan is negative, we scan again in 3 months. The immune system often finds the cancer before the radiologist can see it on a CT scan.

4. Seronegative Autoimmune Encephalitis

This is the challenge of 2026. Some patients have all the signs: inflammation in the spinal fluid, response to steroids, and classic MRI changes (glowing temporal lobes). But their antibody panel is negative.

Course Protocol: We treat the patient, not the lab result. If the clinical suspicion is high, we initiate a trial of high-dose steroids. A dramatic improvement confirms the diagnosis retrospectively. We call this "Probable Autoimmune Encephalitis."

Pediatric Allergy and Transition Care

14.1 The Allergic March and Microbiome

The Trajectory of Atopy

The "Allergic March" refers to the natural history of atopic manifestations. It is a time-dependent progression. It typically follows a predictable sequence, although 2026 data suggests more variability than previously thought.

The classic march begins in infancy with Atopic Dermatitis (Eczema). This is often the "entry point" for sensitization. When the skin barrier is compromised, allergens (like peanut protein or dust mites) penetrate the skin rather than entering through the gut. The immune system, seeing these proteins in the wrong location, flags them as threats.

Following eczema, we often see the emergence of Food Allergy. As the child grows into the toddler years, the manifestation shifts toward the respiratory tract, leading to Allergic Rhinitis (hay fever) and eventually Asthma.

Clinical Example: Consider "Leo." At 3 months old, Leo has dry, red patches on his cheeks (eczema). His parents apply diverse creams but don't address the inflammation. Peanut proteins from his father's hands enter Leo's skin through these micro-cracks. By 12 months, Leo eats peanut butter and suffers anaphylaxis. By age 5, Leo develops a chronic runny nose in the spring. By age 7, he is diagnosed with exercise-induced asthma. This is the Allergic March in action.

The "Old Friends" Theory and Hygiene Hypothesis

For decades, we relied on the Hygiene Hypothesis—the idea that our environments were "too clean," leaving the immune system bored and prone to attacking harmless proteins. In 2026, we have refined this into the "Old Friends" Theory (or Biodiversity Hypothesis).

It is not about being "dirty" in the sense of leaving trash around. It is about the loss of specific, ancestral microbial partners. We co-evolved with commensal bacteria, helminths (worms), and environmental microbiota found in soil and animals. These organisms taught our immune systems tolerance. They stimulated T-regulatory cells (T-regs), the peacekeepers of the immune system.

Without these "Old Friends" due to urbanization, antibiotics, and sterile diets, our T-regs are underactive. The immune system loses its brakes and overreacts to pollen, milk, and pets.

The Microbiome: The Inner Ecosystem

The gut microbiome is the engine room of immune tolerance. By 2026, we understand that "dysbiosis" (an imbalance of gut bacteria) in the first 1000 days of life is a critical risk factor for allergy.

Key players include bacteria like Bifidobacterium and Lactobacillus, but newer research highlights the importance of butyrate-producing bacteria like Faecalibacterium prausnitzii. These bacteria ferment dietary fiber into Short-Chain Fatty Acids (SCFAs). SCFAs are chemical messengers that strengthen the gut lining and calm the immune system.

Environmental Exposures affecting the Microbiome:

Mode of Delivery: C-section babies miss the inoculation of vaginal flora, picking up skin flora instead. This alters their initial gut colonization.

Antibiotics: Early and frequent antibiotic use acts like a forest fire in the gut, burning down diverse bacterial communities that may never fully recover.

Diet: Low-fiber, high-sugar diets starve the "good" bacteria, leading to a leaky gut barrier.

Research Insight: Studies comparing children raised on traditional farms with those in urban apartments consistently show that farm children—exposed to stable dust, animals, and raw milk—have lower rates of asthma. Their innate immune systems are "trained" by the diverse microbial environment.

Evidence-Based Prevention Strategies

How do we stop the march? In 2026, prevention is proactive, not reactive.

1. Skin Barrier Protection

We now treat the skin as an immune organ. "Emollients alone" are sometimes insufficient if inflammation is present. The goal is to repair the "brick and wall" structure of the skin. If a child has eczema, aggressive treatment with anti-inflammatory topicals and lipid-rich moisturizers (ceramides) is crucial to close the door to allergen sensitization.

2. Early Dietary Introduction The old advice to "avoid allergens until age 3" is obsolete. Based on landmark

studies (like LEAP and EAT) and refined by 2026 guidelines, we introduce allergens early and often.

High-Risk Infants: For babies with severe eczema or egg allergy, we introduce peanut products (age-appropriate texture) as early as 4-6 months.

Maintenance: It is not enough to feed the allergen once. It must be part of the regular diet (e.g., 2-3 times a week) to maintain tolerance.

14.2 Pediatric Food Allergy Management

Managing Cow's Milk Protein Allergy (CMPA)

Cow's Milk Protein Allergy is one of the most common food allergies in infancy, but it is also one of the most confusing due to its varied presentation.

Types of CMPA:

IgE-Mediated: Rapid onset (minutes to 2 hours). Symptoms include hives, swelling (angioedema), vomiting, and potential anaphylaxis. Diagnosis is supported by Skin Prick Tests (SPT) or specific IgE blood tests.

Non-IgE-Mediated: Delayed onset (hours to days). Symptoms are mostly gastrointestinal: chronic reflux, loose stools, blood or mucus in stool, and intense colic. Diagnosis is clinical—based on an elimination diet and re-challenge.

Clinical Example: A 4-month-old infant, "Sara," presents with blood-streaked stool and eczema. She is exclusively formula-fed. She does not have hives. This is likely Non-IgE CMPA (Proctocolitis). The immediate action is a dietary change, not an Epipen.

Formula Selection: The Hydrolysate vs. Amino Acid Decision

When a formula-fed infant has CMPA, standard formula (intact protein) acts as a poison. We must break the protein down.

Extensively Hydrolyzed Formula (eHF):

Mechanism: The casein and whey proteins are chopped into tiny peptide chains.

Usage: This is the first-line choice for 90% of mild-to-moderate CMPA cases. It retains enough peptide structure to potentially help the immune system build tolerance over time (immunomodulation).

Taste: Often bitter, but infants usually accept it if introduced early.

Amino Acid Formula (AAF):

Mechanism: Contains no protein chains, only free amino acids (the building blocks). It is elemental and strictly non-allergenic.

Usage: Reserved for severe cases.

- Anaphylaxis to milk.
- Eosinophilic Esophagitis (EoE).
- Severe Failure to Thrive.
- Failure to resolve symptoms on eHF after 2-4 weeks.

Cost: Significantly more expensive.

2026 Update – Synbiotics: Modern formulas in 2026 often include synbiotics (a specific prebiotic + probiotic blend). Evidence suggests these do not just treat the symptoms but accelerate the natural outgrowth of the allergy, helping the child return to normal milk sooner.

Growth Monitoring: Preventing Nutritional Rickets

Eliminating milk is risky. Dairy is a primary source of fats, protein, Calcium, and Vitamin D for toddlers. Without careful substitution, allergic children are at high risk for Nutritional Rickets (softening of bones) and Failure to Thrive (poor weight gain).

Management Protocol:

Dietary Review: A dietitian must be involved. "Almond milk" or "Rice milk" are effectively colored water in terms of protein and fat content for a growing toddler. They are unsuitable as primary drinks for children under 2 years.

Fortification: We must ensure the substitute milk is fortified with Calcium and Vitamin D.

Supplementation: Often, separate vitamin drops are required.

Clinical Reality: We often see "calcium hunger" in allergic children—they may crave chalk or drywall (pica) if their dietary calcium is critically low. Regular growth charting is non-negotiable.

Allergy Management in Schools

By the time a child enters school, the management shifts from parental control to community responsibility.

The Action Plan: Every allergic child must have an Anaphylaxis Action Plan (AAP). This document, usually signed by a doctor, includes:

Photo of the child.

Specific allergens.

Clear symptoms of mild vs. severe reactions.

Dosing instructions for epinephrine.

The Environment: Schools in 2026 are moving away from "bans" (which can create a false sense of security) toward "allergy aware" environments.

No Food Sharing Policies: This is more effective than banning peanuts.

Hand Washing: Soap and water (not sanitizer) remove food proteins.

Inclusion: Ensuring the allergic child is not isolated at a "peanut table," which can lead to bullying and anxiety.

Emergency Medication: Epinephrine Autoinjectors (EAIs) must be unlocked and accessible. A delayed administration of epinephrine is the single biggest risk factor for fatality in anaphylaxis. In 2026, many schools stock "generic" supply autoinjectors for children who may have their first reaction at school and have no personal prescription yet.

Conclusion

The field of Allergy and Clinical Immunology in 2026 is defined by precision. We have moved from broad avoidance to active tolerance induction. We understand that the skin and the gut are the training grounds for the immune system.

In managing the Allergic March, our goal is to intervene early—sealing the skin barrier and diversifying the gut microbiome—to halt the progression to asthma. In managing food allergy, we balance safety with nutrition, ensuring that a diagnosis of CMPA does not lead to nutritional deficits or social isolation.

As clinicians and students of this field, your role is to translate this complex biology into practical, empathetic care. You are not just treating an immune response; you are guiding a family through a life-changing diagnosis, ensuring their child can grow, eat, and learn safely.

14.3 Pediatric Immunodeficiency Red Flags

The Challenge: Normal vs. Pathological

Imagine a busy nursery school in Dublin in winter. Every child has a runny nose. Every child seems to be coughing. As a physician, your hardest task isn't diagnosing the sick child; it is distinguishing the pathologically sick child from the normally sick child.

In 2026, we still rely on the foundational principle that "frequency does not always equal pathology." A healthy toddler attending daycare can legitimately suffer 8 to 10 viral respiratory infections a year. This is the "nursery syndrome," and it is annoying for parents, but it is immunologically normal. It is the immune system's gym class—a workout, not a defect.

So, when do we worry? We worry when the infections break the rules.

The SPUR Acronym

To help physicians cut through the noise, we use the SPUR acronym. This is your mental checklist. If a child fits SPUR, they need an immune workup.
S – Severe

Normal infections are annoying; pathological infections are life-threatening.

The Red Flag: A child requiring intravenous (IV) antibiotics for an infection that should have cleared with oral medication.

Example: Consider a 3-year-old named Leo. He gets otitis media (ear infection). Most kids get this. But Leo doesn't just get a red ear; he develops mastoiditis requiring surgery. That is Severe. It suggests his immune system failed to contain a standard pathogen.

P – Persistent

A normal infection has a beginning, a middle, and an end. An immunodeficient infection just lingers.

The Red Flag: A cough that doesn't go away after weeks of treatment, or "failure to thrive" where the child's body is so busy fighting a low-grade war against germs that it has no energy left to grow.

Example: A 6-month-old infant has oral thrush (candidiasis). This is common. But if that thrush persists despite weeks of nystatin treatment and spreads down the esophagus, that is Persistent. It is a hallmark of T-cell defects like Severe Combined Immunodeficiency (SCID).

U – Unusual

This refers to the organism causing the infection. Humans live in a sea of bacteria. We shouldn't get sick from the weak ones.

The Red Flag: Infections caused by opportunistic pathogens like Pneumocystis jirovecii, Aspergillus, or non-tuberculous mycobacteria.

Example: If a 5-year-old presents with pneumonia caused by Serratia marcescens (a bacteria usually found in bathrooms and soil, not lungs), you must stop. Healthy lungs don't let Serratia in. This is Unusual and screams of a phagocyte defect like Chronic Granulomatous Disease (CGD).

R – Recurrent

This is about volume and location.

The Red Flag: Two or more deep-seated infections (like meningitis, osteomyelitis, or sepsis) in a lifetime, or repeated pneumonias in a single year.

Example: A child who has had bacterial meningitis twice by age four. Lightning rarely strikes the same healthy immune system twice in that specific way. This is Recurrent and suggests a defect in the complement system or antibody production.

Vaccine Safety: The 2026 Protocol

One of the first interventions we perform on infants is vaccination. In the context of Primary Immunodeficiency (PID), this is a double-edged sword.

The Golden Rule of 2026: Live vaccines are a "biological stress test" that an immunodeficient infant will fail—often with fatal consequences.

When a child has a suspected T-cell defect (like SCID) or a severe antibody defect, you must never administer a live vaccine. The live virus, though weakened (attenuated) for healthy kids, can replicate unchecked in an immunocompromised host.
1. Rotavirus Vaccine

The Risk: This is an oral live vaccine given very early (2 and 4 months).

The Danger: In an infant with SCID, the vaccine virus can cause severe, prolonged diarrhea leading to failure to thrive and metabolic collapse.

2026 Practice: If there is a family history of immunodeficiency, or if the newborn screening (TREC assay) is pending or abnormal, the Rotavirus vaccine is strictly contraindicated until the immune system is proven competent.

2. BCG (Bacille Calmette-Guérin)

The Risk: Used for Tuberculosis protection.

The Danger: In infants with SCID or Chronic Granulomatous Disease (CGD), the BCG bacteria can disseminate. It doesn't just stay in the arm; it spreads to the bones, liver, and lungs (BCG-osis).

2026 Practice: In Ireland and the UK, we are highly cautious. We do not give BCG to infants with a family history of PID until they have been cleared by an immunologist.

3. MMR (Measles, Mumps, Rubella)

The Risk: A live injectable vaccine.

The Danger: It can cause vaccine-strain measles pneumonia or encephalitis in T-cell deficient patients.

2026 Practice: We wait. For children on immunoglobulin replacement therapy (IgRT), the donor plasma often provides passive protection against measles, making the vaccine less effective anyway. However, the safety risk is the primary driver. We measure CD4 counts and T-cell function before even considering this in a partial deficiency.

14.4 Transition to Adult Services

Specialty CiP 6: The Transition of Care

We now move to one of the most complex phases in a patient's life: the teenage years.

In the 2026 curriculum, Specialty CiP 6 (Capabilities in Practice) is entirely dedicated to this. Why? Because research shows that the period between ages 16 and 24 is the "danger zone" for patients with chronic conditions. Mortality rates spike here.

Why do they spike? Because the patient is firing their parents as managers but hasn't yet hired themselves for the job.

The Adolescent Brain and Immunology

Adolescents are not just "big children." Their brains are rewiring. The reward centers (seeking dopamine) develop faster than the prefrontal cortex (risk assessment).

Risk-Taking: A teenager with a complement deficiency might decide to skip their prophylactic antibiotics because "I feel fine."

Rebellion: A teen with severe allergies might stop carrying their adrenaline auto-injector (EpiPen) because it ruins the line of their skinny jeans or looks "uncool" at a festival.

This is where you, the immunologist, must stop being a prescriber and start being a negotiator.

The "Ready Steady Go" Program

To manage this chaos, we use a structured framework called "Ready Steady Go." It is not a single event; it is a process that takes years.

Phase 1: READY (Ages 11–13)

The Goal: Introduction.

The Action: We start talking to the child, not just the parent. We explain what their condition is in simple terms.

The Milestone: The child should know the name of their condition and their medications.

Example: You ask 12-year-old Sean, "Why do you take this yellow pill?" If he says, "Because Mum tells me to," he is not ready. If he says, "To stop the bacteria from hurting my lungs," he is getting there.

Phase 2: STEADY (Ages 14–16)

The Goal: Empowerment.

The Action: We ask the parent to leave the room for the first 5 minutes of the consult. This is crucial. It signals to the teen: You are the patient. I am your doctor.

The Milestone: The teen starts managing their own prescriptions and knows when to call for help. They learn about "lifestyle risks"—alcohol, smoking, and how they interact with their meds.

Phase 3: GO (Ages 16–18)

The Goal: Transfer.

The Action: The teen attends the clinic alone (or leads the consultation with parents silent). We finalize the transfer letter to the adult team.

The Milestone: The "Hello" phase. They meet the adult team before they actually move. This reduces the fear of the unknown. We ensure they know that adult hospitals are different—no colorful murals, no play therapists, just efficient, adult-focused medicine.

Vocational Counseling: The Hard Conversations

Part of CiP 6 is having honest, sometimes heartbreaking, conversations about the future. We must guide these young adults toward careers where they can thrive, not just survive.

Military Service: In 2026, most armed forces still strictly exclude candidates with significant PIDs. This is often a blow to young men and women who dream of service. You must break this news gently but firmly early on (around age 14) so they don't build a life plan around an impossibility.

Healthcare Roles: A patient with Common Variable Immunodeficiency (CVID) who is prone to respiratory infections might struggle working in a pediatric ICU where viral loads are high. We might steer them toward pathology, radiology, or research—areas where they help patients without breathing in every circulating flu strain.

Travel and Gaps Years: Adolescents love "gap years." You have to counsel them on where they can safely go. Backpacking through rural areas with limited access to sterile IV equipment or refrigeration for their immunoglobulin is a risk. We help them map out "safe zones"—countries with healthcare systems that recognize their condition.

Future Horizons, Planetary Health, and Professional Development

15.1 Planetary Health and Climate Immunology

The 2026 BSACI curriculum update explicitly recognizes the climate crisis as a health emergency. As immunologists, we are on the front lines. The air our patients breathe is changing chemically and biologically, leading to more aggressive respiratory pathologies.

A. The Changing Aerobiology: Longer Seasons, Potent Pollen

We are no longer facing the "standard" pollen calendars of the early 2000s. The data is clear: rising global temperatures and increased atmospheric CO_2 are fundamentally altering plant biology.

1. The "CO_2 Fertilization" Effect You might recall from basic biology that plants need CO_2 to grow. However, in our current high-carbon atmosphere, we are seeing a "super-charging" effect.

Increased Biomass: Ragweed and birch trees are growing larger and producing significantly more pollen grains per plant than they did twenty years ago.

Higher Allergenicity: This is the critical clinical point. Research indicates that pollen grains grown under high CO_2 concentrations contain higher levels of allergenic proteins (like Amb a 1 in ragweed). The pollen is not just more abundant; it is more potent.

Extended Duration: The 2026 aerobiological data suggests the pollen season has lengthened by an average of 0.9 days per year over the last two decades. In the UK, we are seeing the birch season start earlier in the spring (due to warmer Februaries) and the grass season extend later into the autumn.

Clinical Implication: Patients who previously reported symptoms only in June and July are now presenting from April through September. You must adjust your history-taking to account for these "creeping" seasons. Do not dismiss "hay fever" symptoms in early March or late September as viral infections without considering the altered pollen window.

B. Thunderstorm Asthma: A Climate-Driven Emergency

Once considered a rare curiosity, "Thunderstorm Asthma" is now a core part of emergency planning in the UK and Australia.

The Mechanism It is a perfect storm of aerobiology and meteorology.

High Pollen Load: It typically happens on days with high grass pollen counts (usually Rye grass).

The Storm: A thunderstorm develops. The updrafts suck whole pollen grains into the clouds.

Moisture Shock: Inside the high-humidity clouds, the pollen grains absorb water, swell, and rupture.

The Release: Instead of a single large grain (approx. 35 microns) that gets trapped in the nose, the rupture releases thousands of tiny starch granules (0.5–2.5 microns).

Inhalation: Strong downdrafts push these tiny particles to ground level. Because they are so small, patients inhale them deep into the lower airways (bronchioles), bypassing the nasal filter.

Risk Stratification (2026 Guidelines) The profile of the "Thunderstorm Asthma" patient is specific. It is often not the severe asthmatic.

Primary Risk: Patients with Seasonal Allergic Rhinitis (Hay Fever) who are sensitized to Rye grass, even those with no prior history of asthma.

Secondary Risk: Patients with poorly controlled asthma who are not using preventer medication.

Prevention Strategy

Education: Patients with severe hay fever must be warned that thunderstorms during pollen season are dangerous. They should stay indoors with windows closed during the wind gusts preceding a storm.

Pharmacology: The BSACI emphasizes that "Hay Fever is a lower-airway risk factor." Aggressive management of rhinitis with intranasal corticosteroids is protective.

C. Sustainable Clinical Practice: The "Green" Imperative

The NHS has committed to net-zero targets, and Allergy departments are major contributors to the carbon footprint, primarily through prescriptions.

1. The Inhaler Transition (MDI to DPI) This is the single most impactful change you can make as a clinician.

The Problem: Metered Dose Inhalers (MDIs) use hydrofluoroalkane (HFA) propellants. These are potent greenhouse gases. A typical MDI has the carbon footprint equivalent to driving a car for 175 miles.

The Solution: Dry Powder Inhalers (DPIs) have no propellant. Their footprint is roughly 1/20th of an MDI (equivalent to driving just 4 miles).

2026 Data: Recent studies (e.g., South Tyrol analysis) show that MDIs contribute ~1000 tonnes of CO_2eq annually in small regions, while DPIs contribute <55 tonnes.

Clinical Pearl: Most adult patients can generate the inspiratory flow required for a DPI. Switching a patient from Ventolin (MDI) to a Salamol (MDI with lower carbon) or, better yet, a DPI specifically, is a high-impact climate action. However, patient safety comes first. If a child or elderly patient cannot use a DPI effectively, the MDI remains the correct choice.

2. The "Green Endoscopy" and Clinic Model

Waste Reduction: We are moving away from single-use plastics in skin prick testing where possible, though hygiene remains paramount.

Green Endoscopy: For our rhinology and immunology colleagues, this involves using endoscopes with reusable components, LED light sources to reduce energy, and strict recycling protocols for packaging.

Digital First: Reducing patient travel is a key sustainability metric. A video consultation for a routine follow-up saves the carbon emissions of a car or bus journey. This links directly to our next topic.

15.2 Digital Health and Artificial Intelligence

We are transitioning from an era of reactive medicine (treating the attack) to predictive medicine (preventing the attack), powered by data.

A. AI in Predictive Modeling and Stratification

Artificial Intelligence in 2026 is not about "robots replacing doctors"; it is about "algorithms enhancing insight."

1. Phenotyping and Precision Medicine Asthma and Urticaria are not single diseases; they are umbrellas covering multiple "endotypes."

The AI Role: Machine learning algorithms can analyze vast datasets—blood biomarkers (eosinophils, IgE), genetic markers, and clinical history—to predict which patients will respond to expensive biologic therapies (like anti-IL-5 or anti-IgE).

Example: In pediatric asthma, AI tools analyzing Electronic Health Records (EHRs) have demonstrated 92% accuracy in diagnosing asthma, significantly outperforming traditional clinical scoring methods (85%). This helps prevent misdiagnosis and inappropriate steroid use.

2. The Tolerance Induction Program (TIP) Innovations like those seen at the Food Allergy Institute utilize AI to revolutionize food allergy treatment. Instead of risky "trial and error" food challenges, AI models analyze thousands of data points to predict reaction thresholds. This allows for the creation of hyper-personalized dosing schedules for immunotherapy, ensuring safety and improving the likelihood of remission.

B. Big Data: The National Registries

Data is the currency of modern immunology. In the UK, we have moved towards centralized, robust data collection.

The UK PIN / UKPID Registry Formerly separate entities, the consolidation of immunology registries has created a powerful tool for research.

What it is: A centralized database collecting genetic and clinical data on patients with Primary Immunodeficiencies (PID) and Secondary Antibody Deficiencies.

Why it matters: Rare diseases are hard to study. By pooling data from 38+ NHS trusts, we can identify trends, track the efficacy of immunoglobulin replacement therapies, and spot "red flags" for malignancy earlier than any single clinician could.

The "Missing" Data (2025/2026 Context) A critical 2025 report by Allergy UK highlighted a major gap: nearly 80% of Integrated Care Boards (ICBs) could not accurately track allergy patients in their region. This has driven the push for a National Allergy Register embedded within the NHS Single Patient Record (SPR).

Your Role: As a trainee, you must ensure accurate coding. "Allergy NOS" (Not Otherwise Specified) is a useless code. Precise coding (e.g., "Anaphylaxis to Peanut") allows these national datasets to function, directly influencing funding and service commissioning.

C. Digital Therapeutics (DTx) in the NHS

As of January 2026, NICE (The National Institute for Health and Care Excellence) has formally recommended specific digital platforms for use in the NHS. This is a game-changer.

1. The "Prescribable" App We now have eight digital platforms (e.g., Asthmahub, AsthmaTuner, Digital Health Passport) recommended for evidence generation.

Functionality: These are not just "diaries." They connect to smart inhalers via Bluetooth. They track usage, monitor local air quality, and provide a dynamic Asthma Action Plan that updates based on symptoms.

The "Smart" Inhaler: If a patient uses their reliever inhaler more than three times in a week, the app alerts them and (with consent) their GP. This closes the loop between patient and provider.

2. AI in Diagnostics: Spirometry Spirometry interpretation can be variable depending on the skill of the operator.

New Tech: NICE has recommended ArtiQ.Spiro for NHS use. This AI software reviews the spirogram curves in real-time. It validates the quality of the blow (reducing the need for repeat visits) and offers an interpretive suggestion (e.g., "Obstructive pattern with reversibility"). This democratizes high-quality diagnostics, allowing accurate testing in primary care hubs rather than just specialist centers.

Section 1: Global Health and Disparities (Module 15.3)

Immunology is a global discipline. However, the benefits of immunological science are not shared equally. In 2026, the disparity in access to life-changing therapies remains the single greatest ethical challenge in our field.

The Inequality of Access: Biologics and Immunoglobulins

Modern immunology relies heavily on high-cost therapies. Biologics (monoclonal antibodies) and Immunoglobulin (Ig) replacement therapies are standard of care in high-income nations. They allow patients with Primary Immunodeficiencies (PID) or severe atopic disease to live near-normal lives.

However, a "zip code lottery" exists on a global scale.

The Supply Chain Gap: In many regions of the Global South, the cold-chain logistics required for storing intravenous immunoglobulins (IVIg) are fragile. A patient in a remote rural clinic often cannot access the same plasma-derived products as a patient in a metropolitan center in Europe.

The Cost Barrier: Biologics targeting specific pathways (like anti-IL-4/13 or anti-IgE) remain prohibitively expensive without robust national health insurance.

Example in Practice: Consider a patient with Common Variable Immunodeficiency (CVID). In the UK or Ireland, they receive regular subcutaneous Ig (SCIg) at home. In a resource-poor setting, this same patient might rely on prophylactic antibiotics alone because Ig therapy is unavailable. This leads to preventable bronchiectasis and early mortality. As ACI physicians, we must advocate for "Access to Medicines" initiatives and support biosimilar adoption to lower costs.

Migration Health: The Mimics of Immunodeficiency

Migration is a defining feature of the 2020s. People move due to climate change, conflict, and economic necessity. This movement brings specific challenges to the immunology clinic.

When a migrant patient presents with recurrent infections, the ACI physician must pause. We must not immediately assume a genetic immunodeficiency. We must first rule out "infectious mimics."

Tuberculosis (TB): TB can suppress the immune system and mimic chronic granulomatous disease.

HIV: Advanced HIV infection destroys CD4+ T cells, creating a phenotype identical to severe combined immunodeficiency (SCID) or idiopathic CD4 lymphocytopenia.

Parasitic Loads: Chronic helminth infections can skew the immune response (driving high IgE and eosinophilia), mimicking severe allergy or Hyper-IgE syndromes.

Deep Dive Analysis: The 2026 curriculum emphasizes "Geographic History Taking." You cannot diagnose a fever of unknown origin without knowing the patient's migration route. Did they pass through a region endemic for Leishmaniasis? Did they spend time in crowded camps where TB transmission is high? Screening for these secondary causes is mandatory before embarking on expensive genetic sequencing for primary defects.
International Collaboration

No nation solves these problems alone. The role of international bodies—specifically the European Academy of Allergy and Clinical Immunology (EAACI) and the World Allergy Organization (WAO)—is crucial.

These bodies provide:

Standardized Guidelines: Ensuring that a diagnosis of anaphylaxis means the same thing in Dublin as it does in Dakar.

Registry Data: Pooling rare disease data across borders to understand outcomes better.

Advocacy: Lobbying the WHO to keep essential immunological drugs on the Model List of Essential Medicines.

Section 2: Professional Development and the ACICE (Module 15.4)

The transition from a trainee (Registrar) to a Consultant is a shift in mindset. It is the move from "asking for approval" to "making the final call." Module 15.4 is the bridge to this independence.

The ACICE: Proving Competence

The Allergy and Clinical Immunology Certificate Examination (ACICE) is the final hurdle. It is not just a test of memory. It is a test of judgment.

The Blueprint: The exam blueprint covers the entire spectrum of the specialty. It weighs heavily on clinical application rather than obscure basic science. Candidates must demonstrate they can manage common conditions (asthma, urticaria) perfectly and rare conditions (hereditary angioedema) safely.

Mastering the SAQ (Short Answer Question): The SAQ is where many candidates struggle. In 2026, the marking algorithms favor precision over verbosity.

Bad Answer: "I would check bloods to see immune levels." (Too vague).

Good Answer: "I would quantify Serum Immunoglobulins (IgG, IgA, IgM) and assess functional specific antibody responses to Tetanus and Pneumococcus." (Precise, actionable).

Strategies for success involve practicing "time-pressured synthesis." You must read a complex clinical vignette and extract the three most critical management steps within minutes.

Lifelong Learning: Revalidation and CPD

Passing the exam is not the end. It is the beginning of Lifelong Learning. In 2026, the medical landscape changes too fast to rely on old knowledge.

Revalidation: Every five years, a Consultant must prove they are still fit to practice. This involves:

Patient Feedback: Are you communicating clearly?

Colleague Multi-Source Feedback (MSF): Do you work well in the multidisciplinary team (MDT)?

Clinical Audit: Are your patient outcomes matching national standards?

Continuing Professional Development (CPD): You must accumulate credits annually. This ensures you stay updated on the latest biologic targets or changes in vaccination schedules. If you stop learning in immunology,

you become dangerous to your patients within three years.
Section 3: Specialty Capabilities in Practice (CiPs)

The curriculum measures progress not just by time served, but by "Capabilities in Practice" (CiPs). These are the high-level outcomes of training. By the time you reach CCT (Certificate of Completion of Training), you must operate at Level 4: Unsupervised.

Let us analyze the six critical CiPs defined in Table 1.
1. Allergy Services (Level 4)

This goes beyond treating a runny nose. It involves managing the service itself. Can you set up a drug allergy clinic from scratch? Can you write the business case to hire a specialist nurse?

Example: A Level 4 trainee does not just prescribe an EpiPen. They organize the hospital's anaphylaxis policy, train the emergency department staff, and audit the outcomes of adrenaline administration.

2. Immunology Services (Level 4)

You must run a diagnostic immunology service. This includes interpreting complex laboratory data and liaising with the lab scientists.

Example: When the lab reports a "monoclonal band" in the blood, the Level 4 physician knows exactly how to investigate for Myeloma vs. MGUS without needing a hematologist's hand-holding initially.

3. Diagnostic Advice (Level 4)

Colleagues from other specialties will call you. They will ask, "This patient has low lymphocytes, what do I do?"

The Skill: You must provide clear, safe advice on the limitations of tests. You must stop colleagues from ordering "fishing expedition" tests that yield confusing false positives. You become the gatekeeper of rational diagnostics.

4. Systemic Disease (Level 4)

Immunology is the glue between specialties. We support Rheumatology (autoimmunity), Infectious Disease (host defense), and Respiratory medicine.

Example: In a case of systemic vasculitis, the Immunologist interprets the ANCA results and advises on the risk of immunosuppression, while the Renal team manages the kidney failure. This requires high-level diplomatic and clinical communication skills.

5. Therapeutics (Level 4)

This is the delivery of immune-mediated interventions. It covers the spectrum from Desensitization (making someone tolerant) to Immunosuppression (stopping an attack).

Key Competency: You must be able to manage the complications of these powerful drugs. If a patient on a biologic develops a severe fungal infection, you must know how to adjust the therapy immediately.

6. Transition (Level 4)

Adolescents are not just small adults. They are a unique psychological and physiological group. Transitioning a teenager with severe food allergies or PID from pediatric to adult care is a "danger zone." Adherence to medication often drops during this time.

The Goal: A seamless handover where the young adult takes ownership of their health.

Section 4: Practical Procedures Logbook

Theory is useless without technical skill. Table 2 outlines the progression of practical procedures. The 2026 curriculum emphasizes a clear trajectory: Supervised -> Competent -> Expert.

Skin Prick Testing (SPT)

Status at CCT: Expert/Trainer.

Analysis: By the end of training, you don't just do the test. You teach it. You must know the physics of the lancet, the stability of the extracts, and how to interpret a wheal in a patient with dermographism.

High-Risk Provocations (Drug & Food)

Status at CCT: Competent.

The Risk: These are "live" experiments. You are giving a patient something that could kill them to prove they are not allergic.

Progression: In ST3 (early training), you watch a consultant do it. By ST6, you are running the challenge. You are the one deciding to stop the test because the patient gave a single cough, anticipating the anaphylaxis before it becomes critical.

Desensitization (Drug)

Status at CCT: Competent.

Context: This is often used for chemotherapy or antibiotics (e.g., Aspirin desensitization for cardiac patients). It is high-stakes medicine. The logbook ensures you have performed enough of these under supervision to handle the inevitable reactions calmly.

Laboratory & Physical Skills

Spirometry & FeNO: Competent/Maintain. These are essential for monitoring asthma.

Anterior Rhinoscopy: Competent/Maintain. You must be able to look inside the nose to differentiate allergic rhinitis from polyps or structural deviation.

About Author

Azhar ul Haque Sario is a bestselling author and data scientist with a remarkable record of achievement. This Cambridge alumnus brings a wealth of knowledge to his work, holding an MBA (SZABIST), ACCA (Knowledge Level - FTMS College Malaysia and London College of Accountancy, London), BBA, and several Google certifications, including specializations in Google Data Analytics, Google Digital Marketing & E-commerce, and Google Project Management.

With ten years of business experience, Azhar combines practical expertise with his impressive academic background to craft insightful books. His prolific writing has resulted in an astounding 2810 published titles, earning him the record for the maximum Kindle editions and paperback books published by an individual author in one year, awarded by Asia Books of Records in 2024.

ORCID: https://orcid.org/0009-0004-8629-830X
Azhar.sario@hotmail.co.uk
https://www.linkedin.com/in/azharulhaquesario/

www.ingramcontent.com/pod-product-compliance
Lightning Source LLC
Chambersburg PA
CBHW031343230926
51848CB00002B/370
* 9 7 8 3 3 8 4 8 0 7 8 2 3 *